Dental Implants and Oral Microbiome Dysbiosis

Prasanna Neelakantan
Adline Princy Solomon
Editors

Dental Implants and Oral Microbiome Dysbiosis

An Interdisciplinary Perspective

Springer

Editors
Prasanna Neelakantan
Faculty of Dentistry
The University of Hong Kong
Hong Kong, Hong Kong

Adline Princy Solomon
SASTRA University
Thanjavur, Tamil Nadu, India

ISBN 978-3-030-99013-8 ISBN 978-3-030-99014-5 (eBook)
https://doi.org/10.1007/978-3-030-99014-5

This Springer imprint is published by the registered company Springer Nature Switzerland AG
The registered company address is: Gewerbestrasse 11, 6330 Cham, Switzerland

Prasanna Neelakantan dedicates this book to his parents, his little boss Nilan, his big boss Nithya, his mentors (Professor C.V. Subbarao, Professor Kavitha Sanjeev, Professor James Gutmann and Professor Anil Kishen) and all his students—past, present, and future, for helping him strive to be a better educator every day.
Adline Princy Solomon dedicates this book to the magnificent Queens and strong Princesses of her life who are inspiring and adjusting her crown in every walk of life: (Late) Mrs. Saroja Solomon (Mother), Dr. Agnes Princy Solomon (Sister), Mrs. Mary Sebastian (Sister-in-law), San and Tifany (Daughters) and Ms. Sahana Vasudevan (Student).

Foreword

With great pleasure, I pen down the foreword for the book titled "Dental Implants and Oral Microbiome Dysbiosis: An Interdisciplinary Perspective", which gives a comprehensive outlook of engineering and microbiological aspects of implant dentistry. Several experts from different parts of the world have contributed to this masterpiece, making it a unique contribution to implant dentistry. The book covers a broad spectrum from the basics of dental implants, microbial principles to the recent cutting-edge technology of 3D printing. I congratulate the editors and the authors of the chapters for putting together a timely monograph that is relevant from translational research and clinical perspective. I am sure that the readers will gain a broader perspective of understanding implant dentistry through the eyes of a material scientist and microbiologist. I wish this venture every success.

K. S. Rajan
School of Chemical and Biotechnology
SASTRA Deemed University
Thanjavur, Tamil Nadu, India

Preface

Dear readers, we humbly thank you for choosing to read this monograph. Why another text on dental implants?—you may ask. This book is unique in that it integrates basic principles and factors that influence its success and failure from the microbiological standpoint and introduces several futuristic approaches where biomedical sciences must be integrated with engineering disciplines to offer the best for our patients. While there is nothing as good as the natural tooth, its replacement by artificial prosthesis is sometimes inevitable. While dental implants or implants in the broader context have revolutionized medical treatments, they still suffer from key issues that cause treatment failure. This book is a collaborative venture between basic scientists and clinician scientists who are globally reputed in the fields of implantology, microbiology, host–microbiome interactions, and materials science to bring to you a cutting-edge text that is of equal interest to students and clinicians alike. We are certain that this text will serve as an excellent resource material for undergraduates, masters, and research students spreading across the realms of biomedical engineering, dentistry, and microbiology.

This book is systematically organized into six chapters covering the fundamental aspects of dental implant materials to the latest 3D printing technology. The first three chapters cover the three elements of the infection triangle: environment (dental implants), infectious agent (microbiome), and host responses. The opening chapter provides a birds-eye view of various current designs and materials. The shift then changes cogently to how dysbiotic microbiome causes implant failures. To further strengthen the understanding of how the host reacts to such artificial prosthesis and the infections, the third chapter highlights the host responses to dental implants. With this sold background in the understanding of how infections and host immune responses influence implant success, the next chapter dissects the various research models that have been used to study implant infections both in vitro and in vivo. Naturally, the next section is both current and futuristic. "What can we do to make our implant treatments last longer by preventing infections?" is the question we ask, as we describe state-of-the-art and innovative therapies that may be applied to implant surfaces to beneficially modulate the microbiome. Finally, we conclude with a wave that is revolutionizing the medical and dental fields: bespoke prosthetic engineering which can be made possible by 3D printing.

We are incredibly grateful to all the contributors who have offered the best possible scientific content and insights and bringing this book to its current form. We extend our heartfelt gratitude to the leadership at both SASTRA Deemed to be University and the University of Hong Kong for providing the best resources to its scientists. We thank Prof. S. Vaidhyasubramaniam, Vice-Chancellor, SASTRA Deemed to be University, Prof. S. Swaminathan, Dean of Planning and Development, and Prof. K. S. Rajan, Dean of the School of Chemical and Biotechnology, for their constant motivation and support. We owe sincere thanks to the Dean, Professor Thomas Flemmig, Professor Jukka Matinlinna, and the entire scientific community at the University of Hong Kong, specifically the Faculty of Dentistry, which motivates its academics to achieve the best. The authors of the chapters are pioneers and emerging scientists in the field. We are extremely grateful to all the authors who have shared their expertise through these chapters. We thank the editorial team and Springer Nature for their support throughout the process. We acknowledge the SPARC Division of the Ministry of Human Resource and Development, Government of India, which supported this collaboration. Despite all the glory and satisfaction, being an academic scientist is not without its hidden roadblocks. There are sleepless nights, endless thoughts, constant refocusing of attention to balance life—and all this with the quest to provide the best scientific outputs to ultimately benefit the end user—the patients, who are also taxpayers that support all the research, and this requires unwavering dedication. The editors sincerely thank our families and friends that have always stood by our sides and supported us to continue our goals as educators and scientists. We sincerely hope that this book will be an excellent companion to young minds and researchers in understanding the significant aspects of designing robust implants both for dentistry and beyond.

Hong Kong, Hong Kong — Prasanna Neelakantan
Thanjavur, Tamil Nadu, India — Adline Princy Solomon

Contents

1 **Dental Implants: An Overview** 1
Vinay Sivaswamy and Sahana Vasudevan

2 **Microbial Principles of Peri-Implant Infections** 13
Daniel Manoil and Georgios N. Belibasakis

3 **Host Immune Response to Dental Implants** 31
Nagihan Bostanci, Angelika Silberiesen, Kai Bao, and Ali Gurkan

4 **In Vitro and In Vivo Models to Understand Biofilm Implant Infections** 47
Syatirah-Najmi Abdullah and Nicholas S. Jakubovics

5 **Modern Approaches to Biofilm Management on Dental Implants** 61
Vinay Sivaswamy and Prasanna Neelakantan

6 **3D Printing—A Way Forward** 75
Vinay Sivaswamy, Jukka P. Matinlinna, Vinicius Rosa, and Prasanna Neelakantan

Dental Implants: An Overview

1

Vinay Sivaswamy and Sahana Vasudevan

1.1 Medical Implants: An Introduction

An implant is an artificial device that can repair the functions of biologic tissues and organs or provide a support structure for compromised tissue or replace an entire biologic structure that is missing or damaged beyond repair [1]. Since it is an artificial structure, an implant needs to possess the property of biocompatibility, which in turn refers to the ability of materials to remain passive and non-reactive in human biologic tissue. An ideal biocompatible material can even induce the formation of reparative tissue around it and result in a harmonious union of function and form. A material that is not biocompatible results in a foreign body reaction with the implant material recognised as an invader and being rejected in the form of bone resorption or tissue necrosis, corresponding to the tissue housing the implant prostheses [2].

V. Sivaswamy (✉)
Department of Prosthodontics and Implantology, Saveetha Dental College and Hospitals, Saveetha Institute of Medical and Technical Sciences, Saveetha University, Chennai, Tamil Nadu, India
e-mail: vinay.sdc@saveetha.com

S. Vasudevan
Quorum Sensing Laboratory, Centre for Research in Infectious Diseases (CRID), School of Chemical and Biotechnology, SASTRA Deemed to be University, Thanjavur, Tamil Nadu, India

Implants can be used for a variety of applications, the totality of which can be categorised into two broad modalities—Therapeutic and Cosmetic. Therapeutic uses of implants can further be categorised according to the primary purpose of the implant. (1) Support—surgical meshes which could be metallic (titanium) and used for supporting hard tissue following trauma or it could be synthetic (polypropylene, polyethylene terephthalate, polytetrafluoroethylene and the newer polyvinylidene fluoride, a type of nanofibrous mesh that is resistant to hydrolytic degradation and induces neo-angiogenesis). (2) Replacement—artificial heart, artificial heart valve, coronary stent and dental implant. (3) Repair— intraocular lens, intracorneal ring segment, myringotomy tube, cochlear implant, neurostimulation devices, pacemaker, electric implant, intrauterine devices and diaphragm pacers.

Cosmetic uses of implants are, as the name suggests, related to the improvement of appearance for each individual and are performed solely based on everyone's subjective requirement. The various cosmetic uses can be injectable fillers, which could be transplanted fat or synthetic polymers such as calcium hydroxide, polymethylmethacrylate, polycaprolactone, nasal implants, ocular implants, mammary implants and penile implants. The list of prostheses categorised above are some of the most common usage scenarios

P. Neelakantan, A. Princy Solomon (eds.), *Dental Implants and Oral Microbiome Dysbiosis*,
https://doi.org/10.1007/978-3-030-99014-5_1

and is not intended as a definitive list of commercially available implantation modalities.

A newer application for implants involves the transhumanism approach wherein electronic devices are implanted into an individual's biologic tissue to surpass human limitations. This approach has been termed 'Body Hacking' and a few individuals have succeeded in implanting small electronic devices such as RFID chips into their biologic systems. The most notable examples of this application include the electrode array implanted by British scientist Kevin Warwick in the year 2002 and the antenna implant utilised by British artist Neil Harbisson in the year 2005 [3]. Kevin Warwick succeeded in placing a 100-electrode array into his nervous system. The same procedure was implemented in his wife, which in turn enabled the first direct communication between two nervous systems. The antenna implant utilised by Neil Harbisson is claimed to expand his range of colour sensitivity. It should be noted, however, that this application cannot be adequately supported by valid scientific documentation or evidence and is not recommended as a routine treatment modality by any medical professional.

Implants are currently manufactured using metals and polymers in conjunction with various surface treatments to enable their intended effects. The most common metals used for implants are commercially pure titanium (CpTi), titanium alloy, zirconia, titanium–zirconium alloy, tantalum, stainless steel and cobalt–chrome alloy. The most common polymers used for implants are polypropylene, polyamide, polymethylmethacrylate, polyethylene terephthalate, polytetrafluoroethylene, polyhydroxyalkanoates and polyvinylidene fluoride [4, 5]. A comprehensive dissection on materials used for implantology will be expounded further in the following sections of this chapter.

1.2 Dental Implantology

Till the advent of dental implantology, the most common treatment options for replacing missing teeth involved the detrimental reduction of tooth structure for a fixed prosthesis or the provision of extensive acrylic or metal frameworks for a removable prosthesis. The fixed option involved reduction of multiple teeth for replacing a single tooth and necessitates endodontic therapy in case of unfavourable abutment positions. The removable option involved routine removal of the prostheses for hygiene maintenance and the adjustment of the patient towards the optimal protocol of using a removable appliance [6].

The introduction of dental implants by Per Ingvar Branemark marked the commencement of a revolution in the therapeutic approach for the provision of fixed restorations [7]. The concept of a root analogue for anchorage to the underlying bony tissue marked a paradigm shift in the provision of both fixed and removable prostheses for the replacement of missing teeth. This newer concept eliminated the need for the reduction of adjacent teeth for support and provided the advantage of maintaining alveolar bone height wherever the implants are located. Cumulative evidence from scientific literature show that implants are effective as a definitive restoration modality with success rates ranging from 92 to 95%, depending on the span of the restoration [8, 9]. Other advantages of implants include the elimination of incidence of secondary caries, improved bite force and proprioception. It has been observed that patients develop a sense of proprioception and tactility following implant therapy. Many theories have been proposed to explain this occurrence, with current evidence leaning towards the Bonte theory that hypothesises that re-innervation may occur from stimulation by functional loading [10]. The re-established tactile sense also enables the improvement of bite force magnitude in patients [11]. It should be noted, however, that the tactility and proprioception gained around implants do not reach the same magnitude or intensity of natural teeth, with the active tactile threshold value of implants measured three times higher than that of natural teeth [12].

Success rate is a parameter indicating the treatment outcome following a particular therapy, which could be positive or negative. This parameter has been used as a prognostic indicator with multitudes of studies analysing the success rates for various treatment modalities and suggesting a decision tree for corresponding modalities of therapy. Many studies have reported a 92–95% success rate for dental implant therapy in different scenarios. It has been observed that the success rate is inclusive of implants, whose patients have been subject to confounding factors, such as implants placed after the commencement of a study, which are factors to be excluded from the final analysis. The parameter Cumulative Survival Rate (CSR) is a more appropriate indicator since it would remove confounding factors when analysing failure rates. CSRs usually denote a lower value than success rates but are a far more reliable prognostic indicator. Very few studies have analysed the CSR of dental implants and data remains scarce on these values [13].

Even with the data currently available and the plethora of techniques and equipment, accurate prediction of the treatment outcome for every single case is not yet achievable. Factors such as environment, habit, stress and everyone's biologic response render the treatment modality a measure of probability rather than certainty. It may not be feasible to gain control of each of these factors, yet the implant itself could be rendered conducive to functional adaptation to these conditions. Therefore, most studies attempt to identify favourable characteristics of dental implants to achieve universal acceptability. This task is made doubly difficult due to the existence of hundreds of implant manufacturers as well as the variability in methods that are employed to fabricate implants [14]. Despite the heterogeneity, there are several factors in scientific literature demonstrating the ideal features necessary for a dental implant. A dissection of the constituent portions of an implant is, hereafter, necessary for the identification of ideal features for each portion.

1.2.1 Design Aspects of the Dental Implant: The Current Trend

The term 'Dental Implant' refers only to the fixture that is anchored to the bone. The superstructure that supports the crown, or any prostheses, is termed an abutment. A typical endosseous dental implant can be divided into coronal, middle and apical thirds for the sake of description.

Implants were initially manufactured in a cylindrical shape with the same diameter from the coronal to apical aspect. The fixtures currently available commercially are tapered in a sequentially incremental manner in the apical third to simulate the tapered anatomy of a natural root. The taper also allows easier placement into the prepared osteotomy site whereas a parallel-sided fixture would require more force for complete placement and would, in turn, generate greater torque on the alveolar wall. There were concerns, initially, that the taper would reduce the amount of surface area contacting the bone and would thus, result in poorer osseointegration. These concerns were assuaged when scientific literature displayed that there were no significant differences between cylindrical and tapered implants even in poor density bone, denoting that tapered implants could be used in all conditions.

Implants have transitioned from a smooth, non-threaded surface to a roughened threaded surface since the threads serve a dual purpose of increasing the functional surface area as well as aid in favourable force distribution into the supporting bone. The term favourable force distribution is intentionally used here to highlight the fact that bone is strongest against loads of a compressive manner and weaker against oblique loads. The threads in an implant change the direction of force imparted longitudinally along the axis of the fixture into a transverse direction, which is compressive on the bone [6]. Fixtures with various thread geometries have been implemented by commercial manufacturers across the world with each entity claiming superior osseointegration and clinical longevity due to their thread designs. The thread shapes that have been used till date are square (power thread), fixture (V-thread), acme, buttress thread, reverse buttress, vertical slot, rounded power and spiralock designs [15]. Studies on stress concentrations have shown that there is no difference between various designs, and this has been directly observed in clinical practice as well [16–18].

A direct correlation between the quality of osseointegration in different bone densities and thread size has been observed in scientific literature. Larger threads (increased thread depth and thread pitch) have been found to be advantageous when used in the field of penurious bone density, such as in the posterior maxilla or in cases of immediate implant placement after extraction and smaller threads with reduced depth and pitch perform well in cases of moderate to highly dense bone structures [19].

Microthreads in the coronal portion of the fixture have been observed to retain the marginal bone around an implant after loading. Loading of bone is highest at the crestal region since it is the most superior point of contact of the fixture with bone. The crestal region is thus subjected to the highest magnitude of forces around the implant. Consequently, marginal bone catastrophe is expected to occur till the first thread of the implant. Implementation of microthreads serves to transfer these high-intensity loads into transverse compressive stresses, which the anchoring bone can resist in a more efficient manner. Clinical studies have also shown that the presence of microthreads results in reduced crestal bone loss when compared to implants with a non-threaded smooth surface [20–22].

In addition to microthreads, the method known as platform switching can be used for reducing crestal bone. Platform switching was incidentally observed when a narrower abutment was secured to a wider implant platform and resulted in reduced crestal bone loss [23]. Most implants currently implement platform switching by widening the implant platform diameter and employing an abutment with the same diameter as the implant body. The implant platform is, therefore, wider than the implant body and the overlying abutment and provides the effect of platform switching. Current evidence suggests that platform switching is an effective method of reducing crestal bone loss [24–27].

Implant diameter and length have been established as directly correlative to the main stability of the implant fixture. Implant with wider diameters increases the functional surface area by 200% with every 0.25 mm increase in width [6, 28]. Conversely, implants with a width greater than 6 mm result in a phenomenon known as stress shielding [29]. Stress shielding results from the higher elastic modulus of the implant fixture relative to biologic hard tissue. This mismatch results in viscoelastic flexure of bone under loading conditions whereas the stiffer fixture remains resolute and can cause weakening of the bone–implant interface. There is no evidence, however, to establish the incidence of this shielding phenomenon in routine clinical practice [29]. The lack of evidence could be hypothesised to the fact that implants wider than 6 mm are required to a negligible extent since the alveolar bone is very rarely wide enough to accommodate such diameters. Longer implants engage deeper into the anchoring bone and increase the insertion torque values [30, 31]. Areas of minimal bone, such as the posterior maxilla, may not be able to house implants of increased dimensions. In such cases, a shorter implant with roughened surfaces has been observed to provide an acceptable treatment outcome [32, 33].

It is common knowledge that successful osseointegration occurs once bone remodelling is complete along the implant–bone interface [34]. Remodelling usually requires a duration of 3–6 months depending on the bone density, induction of formative strain and presence or absence of contributing factors, such as infection, diabetes, smoking, bisphosphonate therapy, radiotherapy and so forth [25, 35–37]. It has been observed in scientific literature that modifying the surface area of implants by roughening serves to hasten the rate of remodelling and augments the anchorage of bone to implant. This observation has resulted in a vast swath of laboratory and clinical studies focussed on discovering and/or establishing an optimal method to induce surface roughness and the analysis of optimal intensity of surface roughness that promotes maximal bone integration around the implants [18, 38].

An attempt to identify and categorise the optimal roughness level that hastens bone integration was undertaken by Wennerberg et al., who propounded that a roughness level of 1–2 μm was the most advantageous in improving osseointegration [39]. The research group analysed the surface microtopography of implants and arrived at the conclusion that Sa values of 1–2 μm are the optimal height parameter for a dental implant. They categorised implant surface roughness as mild for Sa values less than 1 μm, moderate for Sa values between 1 and 2 μm and maximal roughness for Sa values greater than 2 μm [14]. These findings are at the micrometre level and it is currently observed that certain surface treatments produce alterations at the nanometre level as well, which further influences the remodelling process.

Surface treatments for implants include additive and subtractive methods, sometimes even a combination of both [40]. The subtractive methods include acid etching, sandblasting/grit-blasting and laser etching. Additive methods are titanium plasma spraying, hydroxyapatite plasma spraying, anodic oxidation and sol-gel deposition. To increase the effectiveness, a combination of subtractive and additive methods such as sandblasting and acid etching, sandblasting, acid etching and ion beam assisted deposition are followed.

Most implant manufacturers employ a combination of surface treatment methodologies rather than rely on any single mechanism. The earliest instances of surface modification were titanium plasma spraying and hydroxyapatite plasma spraying. While titanium plasma spray resulted in rough surfaces (Ra values of 4–5 μm), it resulted in a high incidence of complications and marginal bone loss. The hydroxyapatite plasma spray resulted in high initial stability with eventual coat flaking and delamination which resulted in a foreign body reaction and macrophage induced resorption [38]. Thus, these two methods were discontinued, and the other methods listed above were optimised for dental implant surfaces [18, 41]. Table 1.1 briefs different methods that have resulted in enhanced bone apposition on the implant surfaces when compared with untreated surfaces.

Table 1.1 Different surface treatment methods of dental implants currently in use

Surface treatment modality	Brand name for implant	Manufacturer
Acid etching and anodic oxidation	TiUnite	Nobel Biocare
Grit-blasting, dual acid etching and sol–gel method	NanoTite Prevail	Biomet 3i
Sandblasting (alumina) and acid etching	SLA	Straumann
Sandblasting (zirconia) and acid etching	ZLA	Straumann
Sandblasting, acid etching and ion beam assisted deposition	NanoTite	Bicon
Sandblasting with resorbable blast media	Ossean	Intralock
Sandblasting (titanium) and acid etching	Osseospeed	Astratech

With such an emphasis on implant microgeometry and surface alterations, it is logical to assume that the primary stability of an implant would correlate directly with successful treatment outcomes [20, 42]. Primary stability is a measure of the amount of rigid anchorage attained during implant placement. It is measured through insertion torque using manual torque wrenches, implant stability quotient values using resonance frequency analysis [43], and recently, by value of micromotion as advocated by Trisi's research [44, 45]. While primary stability is a good indicator of a successful outcome following stage 1 implant surgery, studies have found that there is no correlation between insertion torque values and implants under loading conditions [46, 47].

These criteria for endosseous dental implants have been sequestered and compiled from stringently curated scientific literature and have proven to be solid indicators for a successful therapeutic outcome. However, the presence of these factors alone may not guarantee a reliable prognosis since the operator's skill in treatment planning, clinical acumen, presence, or absence of endodontic and/or periodontal infections, systemic factors, play a significant contributory part to the successful outcome of an implant restoration.

1.2.2 Biomaterials in Implant Dentistry: A Historical Outlook

Dental implant materials have a long history from using gold in early 2500 BC to advanced functional "smart" materials in the current generation [48]. The successful osseointegration of the dental implant lies in the design and the material which is chosen for the purpose. Several materials such as metals, ceramics, alloys, polymers and glasses were tried and tested for the dental implant application. In addition to osseointegration, biocompatibility and bio functionality are the factors considered important for the dental implant material [49]. Branemark's monumental discovery of "osseointegration" of titanium to the rabbit bone is considered the benchmark till today. From there, the exploration of different materials for the dental implants began with researchers finding biocompatible materials and modifying the materials having a functional role is in steady progress.

Oral environment is one of the dynamic environments with ever-changing temperature, pH, chemical and physical reactions, making it a challenge for the implant to sustain in such conditions. Thus, an "ideal" implant is required to possess biocompatibility, corrosion resistance, modulus elasticity like bone, wear resistance and strength. These properties of the dental materials are classified as bulk and surface properties [49]. While bulk properties deal with strength and stability of the material, surface properties are crucial for effective osseointegration and increased lifetime. Both the bulk and surface properties define the biocompatibility of the material chosen. Bulk properties of the implant material include modulus of elasticity that should be comparable to bone (10–20 Gpa), high tensile strength for functional stability, improved yield strength to prevent fracture and increased hardness and toughness. Surface properties such as surface tension, energy and topography play an important role in successful host–implant contact [50].

Another important factor is the bio-tribological properties that analyse implant performance based on mechanical wear and electrochemical corrosion [51]. Such tribological tests are important to understand the degradation of the material in the oral environments, which directly translates to the success of the implant. In the case of metals and alloys, crack generation, degradation product and ions releases should be accounted to ensure safe clinical outcome of the implant. Hence the success of the dental implant depends on the different aspects of the material ranging from bulk properties to tribological properties [52].

Dental implant materials can be widely classified as metallic and non-metallic materials. Metallic implant materials include metals and its alloys, which are reliable for implant purposes for a long time.

1.2.2.1 Metal and Its Alloy

Titanium possesses a low density and high strength-to-weight ratio in addition to being biocompatible making it a preferred candidate in the field of dental implants since its introduction in 1981. The integrity of the titanium and the ability to osseointegrate is adequate with a survival rate greater than 90% in the long run. The two most widely used titanium alloys are cpTi and Ti-6A1-4V (titanium–aluminium–vanadium alloy) and they both can readily osseointegrate. The cytotoxicity of Ti-6A1-4V is comparable to that of cpTi despite having vanadium and aluminium. The major alloy used is cpTi, which predictably interacts with air or tissue fluids to form a titanium oxide layer and maintains it without corrosion or breakdown in physiological conditions. Interestingly, this oxide layer directs the implant-tissue interaction such as adhesion of osteoblasts and is a key player in determining the success of osseointegration. Given the major roles played by the implant surfaces in promoting biocompatibility, surface modification remains one of the obvious approaches that influences the outcome of the process. Myriad methods are available for modifying the surface with almost all of them aimed at enhancing the roughness of the surface as it would eventually favour the deposition of proteins promoting soft tissue and osseointegration [53].

Zirconium, like titanium, is a transition metal with excellent biophysical properties. However, with respect to survival and success rates its potential in dental implantology is low when compared to titanium [54]. In the case of fine implants that experience high stress, an alloy of titanium and zirconium (TiZr1317) is employed due to the possession of better mechanical properties such as improved elongation and strength when compared to cpTi [55].

The cobalt–chromium (Co–Cr) alloys contain almost 60% of cobalt and carbon is often added to increase the strength of the alloy. Like titanium, chromium forms the chromium oxide layer on its surface that can resist corrosion. The major advantages of Co–Cr alloys are affordability and mechanical properties such as high elastic modulus and strength thereby allowing the production of fine implants with reduced dimensions. Given that chromium and cobalt are allergens, their application cannot be extended to fixed prosthodontics. They are increasingly used in European countries and it is seen as an alternative to nickel–cobalt alloy in the United States [56, 57].

1.2.2.2 Ceramics

Although metal and its alloys have proven to be durable in the oral environment, especially titanium having strong osseointegration characteristics, the limitations of metal-based implants are many—due to the ever-fluctuating pH of the oral environment, they tend to leach and release the metallic ions into the oral environment, which might trigger an allergic response in some individuals [58]. Previous studies show that on average 0.6% of the population tested show an allergic response to the metallic ions [59]. Furthermore, titanium implants have a lower aesthetic likableness as their distinct metallic colour is often visible through the mucosal tissue [60]. Reports of discolouration of the soft tissue around the region of the implant during the use of titanium implant have also been studied [61]. Thus, the need for novel breakthroughs in material science has provided an alternative to the metal-based approach—ceramics. One of the first ceramics that was used in oral implants was Alumina, but its weak mechanical properties have created a strong need for further research in the ceramic of dental implants [62].

The recent developments have shown zirconia to be a very suitable ceramic-based dental implant approach. Zirconia has excellent osseointegration and mechanical properties to titanium [55] and hence has already been adopted into the implant industry. Zirconia has additionally a lower plaque and bacterial adhesion as compared to titanium, which implies lower fouling tendencies of the implant [63]. It does not have the mucosa decolourisation, host immune reaction that is commonly found with titanium implants.

Hydroxyapatite is a calcium phosphate-based bio ceramic material that has garnered a lot of attention from the Dental Restorative Sciences. Hydroxyapatite is the same material that is known to make up natural teeth and bone. Hence, it has excellent biocompatibility and strong osseointegration characteristics. The major use case of hydroxyapatite in dental implantology has been in the form of coating over pre-existing implant materials [64]. This allows the implant to have a biocompatible surface characteristic while retaining the core mechanical structural integrity of the stronger materials. Since it is made up of the same material as the teeth, it is also subject to the demineralisation–remineralisation dynamics of natural teeth. A much more suitable alternative to hydroxyapatite would be fluorapatite, which is much more resistant to the demineralisation effects of low pH oral micro-environment [65].

1.2.2.3 Polymers

The discovery of synthetic polymers was one of the key innovative concepts of the twentieth century that has revolutionised the way of life in the twenty-first century. Although many polymers have been discovered to date, not all of them have strong relevance in the medical industry due to various factors like biocompatibility. Specifically, for dental implants, osseointegration is also a key criterion for choosing the material among many others, and with titanium having well-studied favourable osseointegration characteristics, it has continued to be the material of choice [66]. But the discolouration and allergic reactions still pose a challenge to be overcome. Among many polymers tried for dental implants, including PTFE, PSU, PMMA, one of the most promising polymers in the dental implant industry is PolyEtherEtherKetone (PEEK) [66, 67].

PEEK has many favourable characteristics and is already used in the medical industry in orthopaedic and vertebral surgery [68]. One of the most common problems with titanium implants is the overloading of the bone via the implant through "stress shielding" [69]. The main cause of stress shielding is the difference in the moduli of elasticity of the materials at the implant junction. PEEK does not have the problem of stress shielding as the mechanical properties of PEEK are similar to bone, thereby reducing the risk of damage to the bone [70]. PEEK by itself has poor osseointegration as compared to titanium [71] but can be used to form composites or be used as a substrate for surface coating [72]. Through this, PEEK-composites and coated-PEEK implants seem to be strong contenders for the future of the implant industry [73]. Hybrid ceramic material with the dual certain-polymer network has been marketed by VITA (VITA Zahnfabrik, Germany) under the ENAMIC brand name. Such hybrid materials with properties from the best of both materials are the need of the hour.

1.2.2.4 Smart Biomaterials

The long-term understanding and the use of dental implants being "passive" is replaced with the concept of "active" biomaterials. In general, such "active"/"smart" materials are known to respond to stimuli in a controlled, reproducible and reversible manner [74]. The application of such smart materials ranges from household supplies to automotive components to biomedical applications.

The concept of "Smart" materials is itself inspired from the natural biological systems. It is well known that simple and complex biological pathways function in response to the stimulus from their environment [75]. The same principle is applied in the design and development of smart materials. Depending on the kind of external stimulus which can be physical (light, electric and magnetic fields, temperature, etc.), chemical (analyte concentrations, change in pH, biological fluids, etc.) and mechanical including stress and strain, the "smart" response is determined. The ability to reverse back to its original state is an important property of such smart materials.

The introduction of smart materials in dentistry was nickel–titanium alloys used for orthodontic wires. The properties of super elasticity and shape memory were utilised in root canal treatment. Furthermore, pH responsive composites are well explored as filler composites, which are self-healing in nature with enriched clinical performance. Smart ceramics mainly zirconia are well explored for their application as dental crowns [76].

With respect to dental implants, the smart response is often associated with surface functionalisation of the dental implants [77]. The primary aspect of such functionalisation is the ability to release antimicrobial compounds such as fluorides and antibiotics to prevent infection in the oral cavity. Nanotechnology is the first choice for such functionalisation purposes owing to its versatile properties. Nanoparticle based surface functionalisation proves advantageous in several aspects in terms of drug stability, minimal cytotoxicity, sustained drug release, improved healing and enhanced osseointegration. Researchers have developed active implant coatings with hydroxyapatite having antibiotics [78]. A sustained release of the antibiotics namely ciprofloxacin and gentamicin were observed. Recently, pH responsive titania nanotube arrays (TNT) which release silver nanoparticles was reported [79]. The TNTs were designed to release silver nanoparticles when the oral environment pH becomes acidic. It is well known that acidogenicity and aciduricity are one of the key virulence drivers which promote peri-implantitis. These properties are practically useful in preventing the biofilm formation on the surface of the dental implants. Even though stimuli responsive dental implants are still in the nascent stage of development, it is to be noted that such implants will prove to be useful on a longer run. While designing a "smart" dental implant, infection management, osseointegration and longevity should be the focus.

1.3 Conclusion

Dental implants are the one-stop solution to the missing tooth. Implant material and design form the basis for successful tooth replacement. This chapter gives a brief outlook on the design and material aspects of the dental implants. The current approach to the dental implants holds the promise to restore the function of the missing tooth. But, with an improved understanding of the dynamic oral environment and oral microbiome, there is huge scope for the development of "smart" dental implants.

References

1. Puleo DA, Thomas MV. Implant surfaces. Dent Clin N Am. 2006;50(3):323–38. https://doi.org/10.1016/j.cden.2006.03.001.
2. Ratner, Buddy D. The biocompatibility of implant materials: Elsevier (Host response to biomaterials); 2015.
3. Lee J. Cochlear implantation, enhancements, transhumanism and posthumanism. Some human questions. Sci Eng Ethics. 2016;22(1):67–92. https://doi.org/10.1007/s11948-015-9640-6.
4. Capellato P, Camargo SEA, Sachs D. Biological response to nanosurface modification on metallic biomaterials. Curr Osteoporos Rep. 2020;18(6):790–5. https://doi.org/10.1007/s11914-020-00635-x.
5. Stewart SA, Domínguez-Robles J, Donnelly RF, Larrañeta E. Implantable polymeric drug delivery devices. Classification, manufacture, materials, and clinical applications. Polymers. 2018;10(12) https://doi.org/10.3390/polym10121379.
6. Misch CE. Dental implant prosthetics. 2nd ed. St. Louis, Missouri: Elsevier Mosby; 2015.
7. Abraham CM. A brief historical perspective on dental implants, their surface coatings and treatments. Open Dent J. 2014;8:50–5. https://doi.org/10.2174/1874210601408010050.
8. Abdulmajeed AA, Lim KG, Närhi TO, Cooper LF. Complete-arch implant-supported monolithic zirconia fixed dental prostheses. A systematic review. J Prosthet Dent. 2016;115(6):672–677.e1. https://doi.org/10.1016/j.prosdent.2015.08.025.
9. Al-Sawai A-A, Labib H. Success of immediate loading implants compared to conventionally-loaded implants. A literature review. J Investig Clin Dent. 2016;7(3):217–24. https://doi.org/10.1111/jicd.12152.
10. Jacobs R, van Steenberghe D. From osseoperception to implant-mediated sensory-motor interactions and related clinical implications. J Oral Rehabil. 2006;33(4):282–92. https://doi.org/10.1111/j.1365-2842.2006.01621.x.
11. Mishra SK, Chowdhary R, Chrcanovic BR, Brånemark P-I. Osseoperception in dental implants. A systematic review. J Prosthodont. 2016;25(3):185–95. https://doi.org/10.1111/jopr.12310.
12. Boven GC, Raghoebar GM, Vissink A, Meijer HJA. Improving masticatory performance, bite force, nutritional state and patient's satisfaction with implant overdentures. A systematic review of the literature. J Oral Rehabil. 2015;42(3):220–33. https://doi.org/10.1111/joor.12241.
13. Griggs JA. Dental implants. Dent Clin N Am. 2017;61(4):857–71. https://doi.org/10.1016/j.cden.2017.06.007.
14. Howe M-S, Keys W, Richards D. Long-term (10-year) dental implant survival. A systematic review and sensitivity meta-analysis. J Dent. 2019;84:9–21. https://doi.org/10.1016/j.jdent.2019.03.008.
15. Atieh MA, Alsabeeha N, Duncan WJ. Stability of tapered and parallel-walled dental implants. A systematic review and meta-analysis. Clin Implant Dent Related Res. 2018;20(4):634–45. https://doi.org/10.1111/cid.12623.
16. Eraslan O, Inan O. The effect of thread design on stress distribution in a solid screw implant. A 3D finite element analysis. Clin Oral Investig. 2010;14(4):411–6. https://doi.org/10.1007/s00784-009-0305-1.
17. Ryu H-S, Namgung C, Lee J-H, Lim Y-J. The influence of thread geometry on implant osseointegration under immediate loading. A literature review. J Adv Prosthodont. 2014;6(6):547–54. https://doi.org/10.4047/jap.2014.6.6.547.
18. Wennerberg A, Albrektsson T, Jimbo R. Implant surfaces and their biological and clinical impact. Heidelberg: Springer; 2015.
19. Udomsawat C, Rungsiyakull P, Rungsiyakull C, Khongkhunthian P. Comparative study of stress characteristics in surrounding bone during insertion of dental implants of three different thread designs. A three-dimensional dynamic finite element study. Clin Exp Dent Res. 2019;5(1):26–37. https://doi.org/10.1002/cre2.152.
20. Falco A, Berardini M, Trisi P. Correlation between implant geometry, implant surface, insertion torque, and primary stability. In vitro biomechanical analysis. Int J Oral Maxillofac Implants. 2018;33(4):824–30. https://doi.org/10.11607/jomi.6285.
21. Lovatto ST, Bassani R, Sarkis-Onofre R, Dos Santos MBF. Influence of different implant geometry in clinical longevity and maintenance of marginal bone. A systematic review. J Prosthodont. 2019;28(2):e713–21. https://doi.org/10.1111/jopr.12790.
22. Niu W, Wang P, Zhu S, Liu Z, Ji P. Marginal bone loss around dental implants with and without microthreads in the neck. A systematic review and meta-analysis. J Prosthet Dent. 2017;117(1):34–40. https://doi.org/10.1016/j.prosdent.2016.07.003.
23. Al-Thobity AM, Kutkut A, Almas K. Microthreaded implants and crestal bone loss. A systematic review. J Oral Implantol. 2017;43(2):157–66. https://doi.org/10.1563/aaid-joi-D-16-00170.
24. Aslam A, Ahmed B. Platform-switching to preserve peri-implant bone. A meta-analysis. J Coll Physicians Surg Pak. 2016;26(4):315–9.

25. Di Girolamo M, Calcaterra R, Di Gianfilippo R, Arcuri C, Baggi L. Bone level changes around platform switching and platform matching implants. A systematic review with meta-analysis. Oral Implantol. 2016;9(1):1–10. https://doi.org/10.11138/orl/2016.9.1.001.
26. Macedo JP, Pereira J, Vahey BR, Henriques B, Benfatti CAM, Magini RS, et al. Morse taper dental implants and platform switching. The new paradigm in oral implantology. Eur J Dent. 2016;10(1):148–54. https://doi.org/10.4103/1305-7456.175677.
27. Meloni SM, Lumbau A, Baldoni E, Pisano M, Spano G, Massarelli O, Tallarico M. Platform switching versus regular platform single implants. 5-year post-loading results from a randomised controlled trial. Int J Oral Implantol (Berl). 2020;13(1):43–52.
28. Lago L, da Silva L, Martinez-Silva I, Rilo B. Crestal bone level around tissue-level implants restored with platform matching and bone-level implants restored with platform switching. A 5-year randomized controlled trial. Int J Oral Maxillofac Implants. 2018;33(2):448–56. https://doi.org/10.11607/jomi.6149.
29. Hingsammer L, Pommer B, Hunger S, Stehrer R, Watzek G, Insua A. Influence of implant length and associated parameters upon biomechanical forces in finite element analyses. A systematic review. Implant Dent. 2019;28(3):296–305. https://doi.org/10.1097/ID.0000000000000879.
30. Korabi R, Shemtov-Yona K, Rittel D. On stress/strain shielding and the material stiffness paradigm for dental implants. Clin Implant Dent Relat Res. 2017;19(5):935–43. https://doi.org/10.1111/cid.12509.
31. Lemos CAA, Ferro-Alves ML, Okamoto R, Mendonça MR, Pellizzer EP. Short dental implants versus standard dental implants placed in the posterior jaws. A systematic review and meta-analysis. J Dent. 2016;47:8–17. https://doi.org/10.1016/j.jdent.2016.01.005.
32. Papaspyridakos P, Souza A d, Vazouras K, Gholami H, Pagni S, Weber H-P. Survival rates of short dental implants (≤6 mm) compared with implants longer than 6 mm in posterior jaw areas. A meta-analysis. Clin Oral Implants Res. 2018;29 Suppl 16:8–20. https://doi.org/10.1111/clr.13289.
33. Uehara PN, Matsubara VH, Igai F, Sesma N, Mukai MK, Araujo MG. Short dental implants (≤7mm) versus longer implants in augmented bone area. A meta-analysis of randomized controlled trials. Open Dent J. 2018;12:354–65. https://doi.org/10.2174/1874210601812010354.
34. Javed F, Romanos GE. Role of implant diameter on long-term survival of dental implants placed in posterior maxilla. A systematic review. Clin Oral Investig. 2015;19(1):1–10. https://doi.org/10.1007/s00784-014-1333-z.
35. Gelazius R, Poskevicius L, Sakavicius D, Grimuta V, Juodzbalys G. Dental implant placement in patients on bisphosphonate therapy. A systematic review. J Oral Maxillofac Res. 2018;9(3):e2. https://doi.org/10.5037/jomr.2018.9302.
36. Moraschini V, Barboza E dS P. Success of dental implants in smokers and non-smokers. A systematic review and meta-analysis. Int J Oral Maxillofac Surg. 2016;45(2):205–15. https://doi.org/10.1016/j.ijom.2015.08.996.
37. Naujokat H, Kunzendorf B, Wiltfang J. Dental implants and diabetes mellitus-a systematic review. Int J Implant Dent. 2016;2(1):5. https://doi.org/10.1186/s40729-016-0038-2.
38. Halpern LR, Adams DR. Medically complex dental implant patients. Controversies about systemic disease and dental implant success/survival. Dent Clin N Am. 2021;65(1):1–19. https://doi.org/10.1016/j.cden.2020.08.001.
39. Albrektsson T, Wennerberg A. On osseointegration in relation to implant surfaces. Clin Implant Dent Relat Res. 2019;21(Suppl 1):4–7. https://doi.org/10.1111/cid.12742.
40. Albrektsson T, Wennerberg A. Oral implant surfaces. Part 1—review focusing on topographic and chemical properties of different surfaces and in vivo responses to them. Int J Prosthodont. 2004;17(5):536–43.
41. Smeets R, Stadlinger B, Schwarz F, Beck-Broichsitter B, Jung O, Precht C, et al. Impact of dental implant surface modifications on osseointegration. Biomed Res Int. 2016;2016:6285620. https://doi.org/10.1155/2016/6285620.
42. Greenstein G, Cavallaro J. Implant insertion torque. Its tole in achieving primary stability of restorable dental implants. Compend Contin Educ Dent. 2017;38(2):88–95. quiz 96
43. Lages FS, Douglas-de DW, Costa FO. Relationship between implant stability measurements obtained by insertion torque and resonance frequency analysis. A systematic review. Clin Implant Dent Relat Res. 2018;20(1):26–33. https://doi.org/10.1111/cid.12565.
44. Trisi P, Berardini M, Falco A, Vulpiani MP. Validation of value of actual micromotion as a direct measure of implant micromobility after healing (secondary implant stability). An in vivo histologic and biomechanical study. Clin Oral Implants Res. 2016;27(11):1423–30. https://doi.org/10.1111/clr.12756.
45. Trisi P, Perfetti G, Baldoni E, Berardi D, Colagiovanni M, Scogna G. Implant micromotion is related to peak insertion torque and bone density. Clin Oral Implants Res. 2009;20(5):467–71. https://doi.org/10.1111/j.1600-0501.2008.01679.x.
46. Berardini M, Trisi P, Sinjari B, Rutjes AWS, Caputi S. The effects of high insertion torque versus low insertion torque on marginal bone resorption and implant failure rates. A systematic review with meta-analyses. Implant Dent. 2016;25(4):532–40. https://doi.org/10.1097/ID.0000000000000422.
47. Lemos CAA, Verri FR, Oliveira N, Olavo B d, Cruz RS, Luna G, Jéssica M, da Silva Casado BG, Pellizzer EP. Clinical effect of the high insertion torque on dental implants. A systematic review and meta-analysis. J Prosthet Dent. 2021;126:490. https://doi.org/10.1016/j.prosdent.2020.06.012.
48. Tomasetti BJ, Ewers R. Short implants. Cham: Springer; 2020.

49. Cicciù M, Tallarico M. Dental implant materials. Current state and future perspectives. Materials (Basel). 2021;14(2) https://doi.org/10.3390/ma14020371.
50. Jiang X, Yao Y, Tang W, Han D, Zhang L, Zhao K, et al. Design of dental implants at materials level. An overview. J Biomed Mater Res A. 2020;108(8):1634–61. https://doi.org/10.1002/jbm.a.36931.
51. Kim J-J, Lee J-H, Kim JC, Lee J-B, Yeo I-SL. Biological responses to the transitional area of dental implants. Material- and structure-dependent responses of peri-implant tissue to abutments. Materials (Basel). 2019;13(1) https://doi.org/10.3390/ma13010072.
52. Dini C, Costa RC, Sukotjo C, Takoudis CG, Mathew MT, Barão VAR. Progression of bio-tribocorrosion in implant dentistry. Front Mech Eng. 2020;6:17. https://doi.org/10.3389/fmech.2020.00001.
53. Nicholson JW. Titanium alloys for dental implants. A review. Prosthesis. 2020;2(2):100–16. https://doi.org/10.3390/prosthesis2020011.
54. Depprich R, Naujoks C, Ommerborn M, Schwarz F, Kübler NR, Handschel J. Current findings regarding zirconia implants. Clin Implant Dent Relat Res. 2014;16(1):124–37. https://doi.org/10.1111/j.1708-8208.2012.00454.x.
55. Patil R. Zirconia versus titanium dental implants. A systematic review. J Dent Implant. 2015;5(1):39. https://doi.org/10.4103/0974-6781.154430.
56. Holm C, Morisbak E, Kalfoss T, Dahl JE. In vitro element release and biological aspects of base-metal alloys for metal-ceramic applications. Acta Odontol Scand. 2015;1(2–4):70–5. https://doi.org/10.3109/23337931.2015.1069714.
57. Kassapidou M, Franke SV, Hjalmarsson L, Johansson CB. Cobalt-chromium alloys in fixed prosthodontics in Sweden. Acta Odontol Scand. 2017;3(1):53–62. https://doi.org/10.1080/23337931.2017.1360776.
58. Souza JCM, Apaza-Bedoya K, Benfatti CAM, Silva FS, Henriques B. A comprehensive review on the corrosion pathways of titanium dental implants and their biological adverse effects. Metals. 2020;10(9):1272. https://doi.org/10.3390/met10091272.
59. Sicilia A, Cuesta S, Coma G, Arregui I, Guisasola C, Ruiz E, Maestro A. Titanium allergy in dental implant patients. A clinical study on 1500 consecutive patients. Clin Oral Implants Res. 2008;19(8):823–35. https://doi.org/10.1111/j.1600-0501.2008.01544.x.
60. Cosgarea R, Gasparik C, Dudea D, Culic B, Dannewitz B, Sculean A. Peri-implant soft tissue colour around titanium and zirconia abutments. A prospective randomized controlled clinical study. Clin Oral Implants Res. 2015;26(5):537–44. https://doi.org/10.1111/clr.12440.
61. Thoma DS, Ioannidis A, Cathomen E, Hämmerle CHF, Hüsler J, Jung RE. Discoloration of the peri-implant mucosa caused by zirconia and titanium implants. Int J Periodontics Restorative Dent. 2016;36(1):39–45. https://doi.org/10.11607/prd.2663.
62. Andreiotelli M, Wenz HJ, Kohal R-J. Are ceramic implants a viable alternative to titanium implants? A systematic literature review. Clin Oral Implants Res. 2009;20(Suppl 4):32–47. https://doi.org/10.1111/j.1600-0501.2009.01785.x.
63. Scarano A, Piattelli M, Caputi S, Favero GA, Piattelli A. Bacterial adhesion on commercially pure titanium and zirconium oxide disks. An in vivo human study. J Periodontol. 2004;75(2):292–6. https://doi.org/10.1902/jop.2004.75.2.292.
64. Ong JL, Chan DC. Hydroxyapatite and their use as coatings in dental implants. A review. Crit Rev Biomed Eng. 2000;28(5–6):667–707. https://doi.org/10.1615/CritRevBiomedEng.v28.i56.10.
65. Pajor K, Pajchel L, Kolmas J. Hydroxyapatite and fluorapatite in conservative dentistry and oral implantology—A review. Materials. 2019;12(17) https://doi.org/10.3390/ma12172683.
66. Knaus J, Schaffarczyk D, Cölfen H. On the future design of bio-inspired polyetheretherketone dental implants. Macromol Biosci. 2020;20(1):e1900239. https://doi.org/10.1002/mabi.201900239.
67. Osman RB, Swain MV. A critical review of dental implant materials with an emphasis on titanium versus zirconia. Materials (Basel). 2015;8(3):932–58. https://doi.org/10.3390/ma8030932.
68. Al-Rabab'ah M, Hamadneh W', Alsalem I, Khraisat A, Abu Karaky A. Use of high performance polymers as dental implant abutments and frameworks. A case series report. J Prosthodont. 2019;28(4):365–72. https://doi.org/10.1111/jopr.12639.
69. Nagasawa M, Takano R, Maeda T, Uoshima K. Observation of the bone surrounding an overloaded implant in a novel rat model. Int J Oral Maxillofac Implants. 2013;28(1):109–16. https://doi.org/10.11607/jomi.2388.
70. Mishra S, Chowdhary R. PEEK materials as an alternative to titanium in dental implants. A systematic review. Clin Implant Dent Relat Res. 2019;21(1):208–22. https://doi.org/10.1111/cid.12706.
71. Najeeb S, Bds ZK, Bds SZ, Bds MSZ. Bioactivity and osseointegration of PEEK are inferior to those of titanium. A systematic review. J Oral Implantol. 2016;42(6):512–6. https://doi.org/10.1563/aaid-joi-d-16-00072.
72. Rahmitasari F, Ishida Y, Kurahashi K, Matsuda T, Watanabe M, Ichikawa T. PEEK with reinforced materials and modifications for dental implant applications. Dent J. 2017;5(4) https://doi.org/10.3390/dj5040035.
73. Xie C, Zhang J-F, Li S. Polymer infiltrated ceramic hybrid composites as dental materials. Oral Health Dent Stud. 2018;1(1) https://doi.org/10.31532/OralHealthDentStud.1.1.002.
74. Badami V, Ahuja B. Biosmart materials. Breaking new ground in dentistry. Sci World J. 2014;2014:986912. https://doi.org/10.1155/2014/986912.
75. Jeong B, Gutowska A. Lessons from nature. Stimuli-responsive polymers and their biomedical applica-

tions. Trends Biotechnol. 2002;20(7):305–11. https://doi.org/10.1016/S0167-7799(02)01962-5.
76. Sivakumar P, Naseem I. Biosmart materials the future of dentistry. A review. Int J Contemp Microbiol. 2016;9(10):1737. https://doi.org/10.5958/0974-360X.2016.00350.4.
77. Wieszczycka K, Staszak K, Woźniak-Budych MJ, Litowczenko J, Maciejewska BM, Jurga S. Surface functionalization—The way for advanced applications of smart materials. Coord Chem Rev. 2021;436:213846. https://doi.org/10.1016/j.ccr.2021.213846.
78. Karacan I, Macha IJ, Choi G, Cazalbou S, Ben-Nissan B. Antibiotic containing poly lactic acid/hydroxyapatite biocomposite coatings for dental implant applications. KEM. 2017;758:120–5. https://doi.org/10.4028/www.scientific.net/KEM.758.120.
79. Dong Y, Ye H, Liu Y, Xu L, Wu Z, Hu X, et al. pH dependent silver nanoparticles releasing titanium implant. A novel therapeutic approach to control peri-implant infection. Colloids Surf B Biointerfaces. 2017;158:127–36. https://doi.org/10.1016/j.colsurfb.2017.06.034.

Microbial Principles of Peri-Implant Infections

2

Daniel Manoil and Georgios N. Belibasakis

2.1 Introduction

The advent of osseointegrated dental implants has revolutionized treatment planning in reconstructive dentistry owing to their unparalleled ability to restore masticatory, occlusal and esthetic functions, compared to other conventional treatments. Dental implants are screw-like devices that are surgically inserted into the alveolar bone to replace one or more missing teeth. In order to be functionally loaded with a prosthetic element, dental implants display a transmucosal interface that mediates the transition from the endosseous part to the peri-implant submucosa and the intraoral environment [1]. As such, dental implants exhibit the unique feature, amid other types of endosseous implants, of being partially exposed to a microbial-rich environment, the oral cavity, which naturally renders them prone to biofilm colonization. Not unexpectedly, the increasing number of implants inserted worldwide has coincided with an overall increase in peri-implant infections [2].

Because dental implants are expected to functionally substitute to natural teeth, there is also a tendency to perceive diseases of ailing implants as pathologies analogous to gingivitis and periodontitis [3]. However, as further described in this chapter, the etiopathological basis of these two groups of oral diseases is not entirely the same. Increasing evidence indicates that the peri-implant ecosystem differs from the natural one established in the gingival crevice around the periodontal tissues, reflecting compositionally distinct microbiota [4]. Yet, compositional shifts within this microbiota may set off a vicious cycle between microbial dysbiosis, ecological alterations, and inflammation that eventually leads to the destruction of the implant-supporting tissues. Within this chapter, we describe the microbial and ecological triggers of peri-implant affections, with a particular focus laid on the microbial community-based aspects.

2.2 Epidemiological Aspects of Peri-Implant Infections

Peri-implant infections are categorized according to the extent of the biofilm-induced inflammation within tissues surrounding the implant. If the inflammation remains limited to the peri-implant mucosal tissues, the condition is termed peri-implant mucositis, whereas if the inflammation extends to the underlying bone causing peri-implant osteolysis, the condition is referred to as peri-implantitis [5]. Diagnosis of peri-implant infections primarily relies on the clinical and radiographical signs of the induced inflammatory

D. Manoil (✉) · G. N. Belibasakis
Division of Oral Diseases, Department of Dental Medicine, Karolinska Institute, Huddinge, Sweden
e-mail: Daniel.Manoil@ki.se; George.Belibasakis@ki.se

P. Neelakantan, A. Princy Solomon (eds.), *Dental Implants and Oral Microbiome Dysbiosis*,
https://doi.org/10.1007/978-3-030-99014-5_2

changes. Accordingly, diagnostic criteria for peri-implant mucositis include bleeding on probing (BOP), yet without radiographic signs of crestal bone loss beyond the initial remodeling [6]. In contrast, radiographic evidence of osteolysis, typically appearing as a symmetrical "saucer-shaped" crestal defect around the implant, is central to the diagnosis of peri-implantitis. Clinically, an increased probing pocket depth (PPD), as compared to previous examinations is also indicative of peri-implantitis; however, the angulation, insertion depth, and threads of some implants may render probing challenging [6]. BOP-positive peri-implant sites run a higher probability to be diagnosed with peri-implantitis [7], whereas suppuration appears to be very much limited to peri-implantitis cases [8], and its presence is a good discriminant between health or peri-implant mucositis and actual peri-implantitis [9]. The prevalence of peri-implantitis has been earlier reported at 28–56% of implant-baring patients, or 12–43% of the total number of implants [10], with a weighed mean prevalence later estimated at 22% [11]. Principal reasons accounting for variations in these epidemiological observations are the differences in study periods, case definitions, sampling strategies, and the study protocols used. Overall, about one-third of all patients and one-fifth of all implants will be affected by peri-implantitis [12]. Major risk factors associated with these epidemiological observations include past history of periodontitis, smoking, and diabetes, particularly in the absence of adequate oral hygiene [13–17]. Ill-fitting or ill-designed fixed and cement-retained restorations are also evident factors of local plaque accumulation [12].

2.3 Biogeography of the Oral Environment

The oral environment represents a unique ecosystem, which is both spatially and ecologically diverse. It is bathed in a constant salivary flow produced by three pairs of major salivary glands along with a plethora of minor glands, each of which secretes saliva that differs in protein and mucin content [18, 19]. Most of the cavity is coated by shedding epithelia, forming a keratinized mucosa onto the hard palate and gingiva, whereas nonkeratinized epithelium is covering cheeks, alveolar mucosa, and the underside of the tongue. A specialized mucosa, coarser and presenting densely packed papilla is found on the dorsum of the tongue [20]. In contrast to shedding epithelial surfaces, teeth offer non-shedding hard tissues anchored to the alveolar bone socket by strong connective tissues. The interface between teeth and the gingiva creates a crevice, termed the gingival sulcus, which physiologically contains a nutrient-rich, serum-derived transudate [21]. This spatial diversity generates ecological gradients characterized by varying levels of temperature, redox potential, or pH, as well as local sinks of nutrients with different access to saliva or crevicular fluid. These locally differing conditions represent ecological niches, that is, microenvironments that differently support the growth of the residing microbiota [22].

The oral microbiota, that is, the entire collection of microorganisms that thrives within this ecosystem, is one of the richest of the human body. The domain bacteria vastly dominates the oral microbiota even though archaea, fungi, viruses, and protozoa can also be detected as constituents [23, 24]. Thus far, the Human Oral Microbiome Database (HOMD) has cataloged 16 different bacterial phyla further subdivided into 687 species-level taxa [25]. Within this taxonomic diversity, different phylotypes require different ecological conditions to meet their physiological needs of nutrients, pH, temperature or O_2/CO_2 concentrations [22]. Naturally then, spatial gradients of these conditions determine the biogeographical distribution of microbial communities among the various niches of the oral cavity [26]. In essence, "biogeography" implies that distinct sites are selective for compositionally different microbial communities than those of neighboring sites associated with varying ecological conditions [27]. As such, oral microbial communities behave as "site-specialists" that are found in the highest relative abundance in a preferred (primary) ecological niche [28]. Furthermore, the microbiota established in an ecological niche may display a reciprocal relationship with its immediate environment. Via their proteolytic or oxygen-quenching activities, for instance, microbial communities may actively influence pH levels, redox potential, or nutrient sources over short spatial scales [29]. This remodeling of their closest environment may alter the ecosystem enough to now foster and promote the establishment of other species, thereby shifting the composition of the microbial community [30].

2.4 The Biofilm Lifestyle: Importance of Microbial Co-Aggregation

To resist the constant salivary flow and be able to thrive in their preferred ecological niche, oral communities must adhere onto surfaces and form biofilms [31]. Non-shedding surfaces are ideal for that purpose, as they are readily coated with proteins and glycoproteins of salivary origin that form a thin layer termed the "acquired enamel pellicle" (AEP) [32]. Components of the AEP, such as sialylated mucins, statherins, histatins, cystatins, or proline-rich proteins, provide binding motifs that enable the selective attachment of early colonizing bacterial species that express cognate surface adhesins [31, 33]. Commensal species (i.e., health-associated ones) such as *Streptococcus salivarius, S. mitis, S. gordonii, S. oralis,* or *S. sanguinis* are typical early colonizers that recognize motifs present in the AEP [34]. Just hours following initial bacterial adhesion, so-called *bridging* species that include *Fusobacterium nucleatum* or *Prevotella loescheii*, adhere to these early colonizers, in turn providing the surface receptors for the incremental co-aggregation of late colonizers [35, 36]. These successive intergeneric co-aggregations represent a reproducible process regulated by affinity-depend interactions between species [37, 38]. In addition to anchoring bacteria to a surface, intermicrobial co-aggregation results in an organized juxtaposition of cells that colocates bacteria in proximity to ecologically relevant partner species, thereby enabling gene transfer, facilitating interspecies signaling and promoting mutually beneficial networking ("syntrophy") [39]. Typical examples of syntrophic interactions include obligate anaerobes that co-aggregate with oxygen-consuming species to survive in aerobic environments, or bacteria that benefit from the proteolytic activity of other species for amino acid supplies [40, 41]. Cell–cell contact also promotes the synthesis of an extracellular polymeric substance (EPS) that enhances adhesion to surfaces and creates a protective barrier against environmental stresses [39, 42]. In the oral cavity, co-aggregated bacteria enmeshed in their self-produced extracellular matrix define the "dental plaque," which microbiologically holds the full properties of a biofilm.

2.5 "Quorum Sensing"—Intergeneric Bacterial Communication

Bacteria can communicate without the need of direct cell–cell signaling. This intermicrobial communication system, termed "quorum sensing," relies on the accumulation of secreted signaling molecules in the vicinity of bacterial populations that reach a certain density threshold (quorum). Binding of these molecules to their cognate receptors induces a series of signal transductions that coordinate gene expression in the microbial community [43]. In doing so, quorum sensing endows microbial communities with the ability to synchronize their phenotype in order to establish mutually beneficial interactions between their independent constituent microorganisms and to better respond to environmental cues [44]. In gram-negative bacteria, most quorum signaling molecules were shown to belong to the class of N-acyl homoserine lactones, short acyl chains that easily diffuse across outer membranes [45]. In contrast, small soluble peptides called autoinducers (AI) that bind to membrane-bound receptors are more commonly involved in gram-positive signaling.

In oral microbiology, particular focus was laid on autoinducer-2 (AI-2), as it was shown to act as an intergeneric signaling molecule, and thus to be crucial for the formation of multispecies biofilms as always encountered in the oral ecosystem. It has been observed, for instance, that several oral commensals such as *S. oralis* or *Actinomyces naeslundii* require a mutual induction by AI-2 to efficiently form biofilms together [46]. Local gradients of AI-2 are also an integral element of the pathogenicity of oral communities. Whereas commensals produce and respond to low amounts of AI-2, further aggregation of late colonizers, such as *F. nucleatum*, is associated with increasing AI-2 levels [31, 47]. *F. nucleatum* is indeed an important producer of AI-2, becomes the predominant gram-negative species in oral biofilms shortly after its adhesion, and further co-aggregates with known periodontal pathogens such as *Porphyromonas gingivalis*, *Tannerella forsythia*, or *Treponema denticola* [34, 48]. Therefore, increasing local concentrations of AI-2 may encourage further development of asaccharolytic/proteolytic species that induce a transition toward more pathogenic communities.

2.6 Histological Characteristics of Osseointegrated Dental Implants

To better apprehend the microbial triggers of peri-implant diseases, there is merit at this stage to identify the fundamental histological differences between dental implants and natural teeth. Most dental implants are manufactured out of titanium alloys, and consist of an orally exposed transmucosal smooth-surfaced section, and an endosseous rough-surfaced section [1]. The latter is designed to promote osseointegration, a process during which the implant develops a direct interface with the surrounding bone [49]. Consequently, osseointegrated implants lack the periodontal ligament (PDL), as opposed to natural teeth that are socketed into the alveolus via fibers of the PDL and supracrestal collagen insertions (dento-gingival and -periosteal fibers) [50]. Instead, supracrestal fibers are circumferentially organized around implants to form a fibrous "collar." Figure 2.1 schematically represents the principal histological differences between implants and natural teeth (Fig. 2.1a, b). The resulting peri-implant crevice is deeper than the natural gingival sulcus, a configuration that weakens the physical barrier against bacterial invasion of the peri-implant submucosa, compared to gingival tissues around natural teeth. Furthermore, the absence of PDL reduces the blood supply to supra-periosteal vessels, and consequently limits the availability of immune cells that may extravasate to tackle early stages of a potential infection [51]. Together, these factors may render dental implants more susceptible to endogenous oral infections [3, 49, 52].

2.7 The Peri-Implant Ecosystem: From Symbiosis to Dysbiosis and Inflammation

Upon insertion, dental implants offer a pristine, non-shedding surface onto which a salivary pellicle rapidly adsorbs, just like with natural teeth. Yet, the composition of pellicles adsorbed onto titanium or enamel surfaces display molecular differences [53]. Whereas titanium-formed pellicles comprise common elements with enamel-acquired pellicles, such as proline-rich proteins, secretory IgA, α-amylase, and high molecular weight mucins, they appear to lack low molecular weight mucins and cystatins [53]. It remains unclear to what extent these differences may affect the bacterial recognition of the pellicle. Although it has been observed that the dynamics of bacterial colonization on implant surfaces are initially slower than on natural teeth [54], the sequence and composition of early colonizing communities appear unaffected [55, 56].

Early colonizers adhere to implant surfaces within 30 min following implant insertion [57] and evolve toward the formation of organized biofilm communities in the next 2 weeks [54]. The composition of the microbial communities that have colonized the peri-implant niche at this stage resembles those of healthy neighboring gingival sulci [58], with nonetheless lower taxonomic diversity [59]. This microbiota may coexist in symbiosis with the host and be compatible with peri-implant health. However, factors that promote biofilm growth, such as poor oral hygiene, induce inflammatory changes within the peri-implant sul-

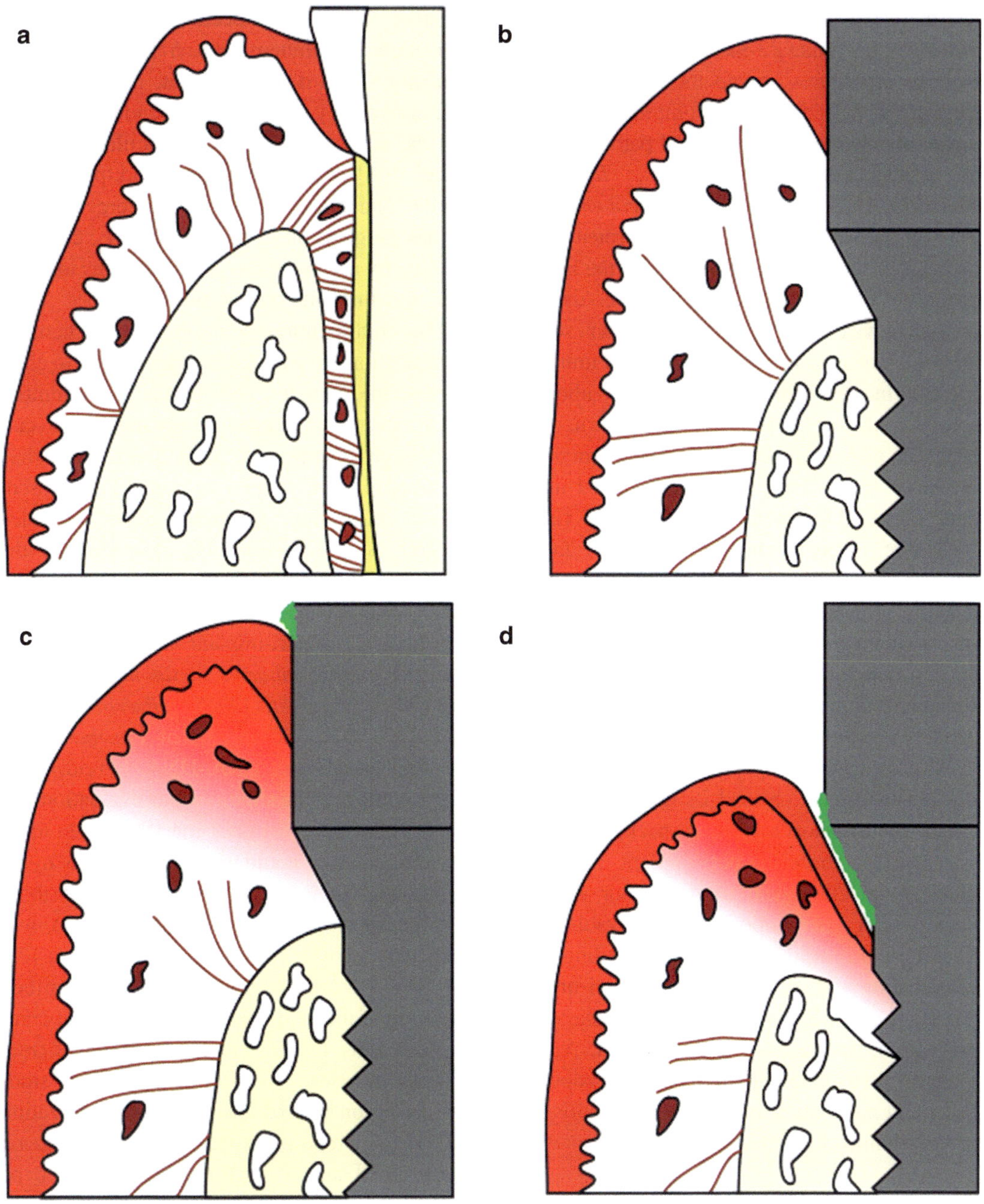

Fig. 2.1 Schematic representation comparing periodontal and peri-implant tissues. A healthy periodontal and peri-implant situation is depicted in (**a**) and (**b**) respectively. The absence of periodontal ligament and direct contact between the bone and the implant surface is shown. The effect of biofilm accumulation (marked green) onto the implant surface is depicted in (**c**) and (**d**). In peri-implant mucositis, the inflammation is restricted to the peri-implant submucosa, without evidence of bone destruction (**c**). During the progression to peri-implantitis, the extent of inflammation results in the destruction of the implant-supporting bone (**d**). (Source: Belibasakis et al. [52]. Reproduced with permission from Springer Nature under the license number 4984180931936)

cus that challenge the equilibrium of this ecosystem. If uncontrolled, inflammation rapidly triggers ecological shifts that lead to dysbiotic transitions in microbial communities. Inflammation increases the exudation of peri-implant crevicular fluid, which creates a protein-rich environment that fosters the establishment of proteolytic species [3]. Evidence shows that a 3-weeks interruption of oral hygiene procedures around the implant is sufficient to shift peri-implant communities toward higher abundances of periodontal pathogens such as species of *Porphyromonas*, *Tannerella*, *Prevotella*, *Fretibacterium*, or *Treponema* [60]. Through the expression of various proteases and hydrolases, these species further alter the nutrient conditions of their ecological niche (i.e., the peri-implant crevice), induce tissue breakdown, subvert the complement system, and impair host immunity [61, 62]. Increased abundance of these pathogenic species in the peri-implant crevice, in turn, correlates with increased secretion of pro-inflammatory cytokines [60]. These microbial-induced alterations collectively set off a self-feeding vicious cycle that enhances and maintains peri-implant inflammation. Whereas this inflammation initially remains limited to the peri-implant submucosa (peri-implant mucositis), its persistence leads to the destruction of underlying connective and bone structures, ultimately jeopardizing implant functionality (peri-implantitis) (Fig. 2.1c, d) [5].

Although the propensity to develop peri-implant inflammation, and its degree, are influenced by the host's genetic background and systemic condition, the peri-implant microbiota remains the etiological trigger factor and one upon which intervention is conceivable [15]. Therefore, a comprehensive understanding of its composition and shifts that lead to peri-implant disease is paramount to improve early diagnosis, prevention, and treatment approaches. All the more so that inflammatory tissue breakdown is faster and more extensive in peri-implantitis than in periodontitis [3, 63].

2.8 Early Work on Peri-Implant Microbial Communities

Initial attempts to characterize the microbial communities associated with peri-implant infections relied on anaerobic culture-based techniques and phase-contrast microscopy [64, 65]. These early reports identified mainly gram-positive cocci, nonmotile bacilli, and few gram-negative anaerobic species in the healthy peri-implant submucosa [66, 67]. The microbial transition toward peri-implant mucositis was characterized by an increased abundance of cocci and the emergence of motile bacilli and spirochetes [68]. Gram-negative, black-pigmented, motile, and anaerobic species emerged during further progression to peri-implantitis, certainly fostered by the lower oxygen conditions in deepened peri-implant pockets [69].

Microbial culture, isolation, and biochemical identification are painstaking approaches to characterize the complex peri-implant communities and are massively limited by our inability to culture "as-yet-uncultivated" taxa, that is, more than one-third of oral species to date [25]. Closed-ended molecular methods have provided researchers with faster ways of evaluating the complexity of microbial communities based on the detection of species-specific genes. Typically, PCR analyses of peri-implant samples frequently detected *Aggregatibacter actinomycetemcomitans* [70], *P. gingivalis* [70, 71], *Prevotella intermedia* [70, 72], and species of *Fusobacterium* [72]. Checkerboard DNA–DNA hybridization analysis allowed the simultaneous evaluation of a bigger set of bacterial taxa; the DNA from up to 40 selected taxa could be arrayed on a nylon membrane. To evaluate the presence of these selected species in a given sample, DNA was extracted and hybridized with the membrane [73, 74]. Such DNA-checkerboard methods identified members of the "red complex" cluster, that comprises *P. gingivalis*, *T. forsythia* and *T. denticola*, to thrive in cases of peri-implantitis. Other studies relying on fluorescence *in situ* hybridization (FISH) also reported species from *Treponema* groups I–III and *Synergistetes* cluster A to be typically associated with peri-implantitis communities [75]. Figure 2.2 displays representative FISH observations of oral Spirochaetes and Synergistetes in peri-implantitis-associated submucosal biofilms (Fig. 2.2a–d).

Taken together, closed-ended molecular approaches mostly pointed out microbial similarities between peri-implant infections and gingivitis or periodontitis. The only microbiological differences that seemed to emerge, came

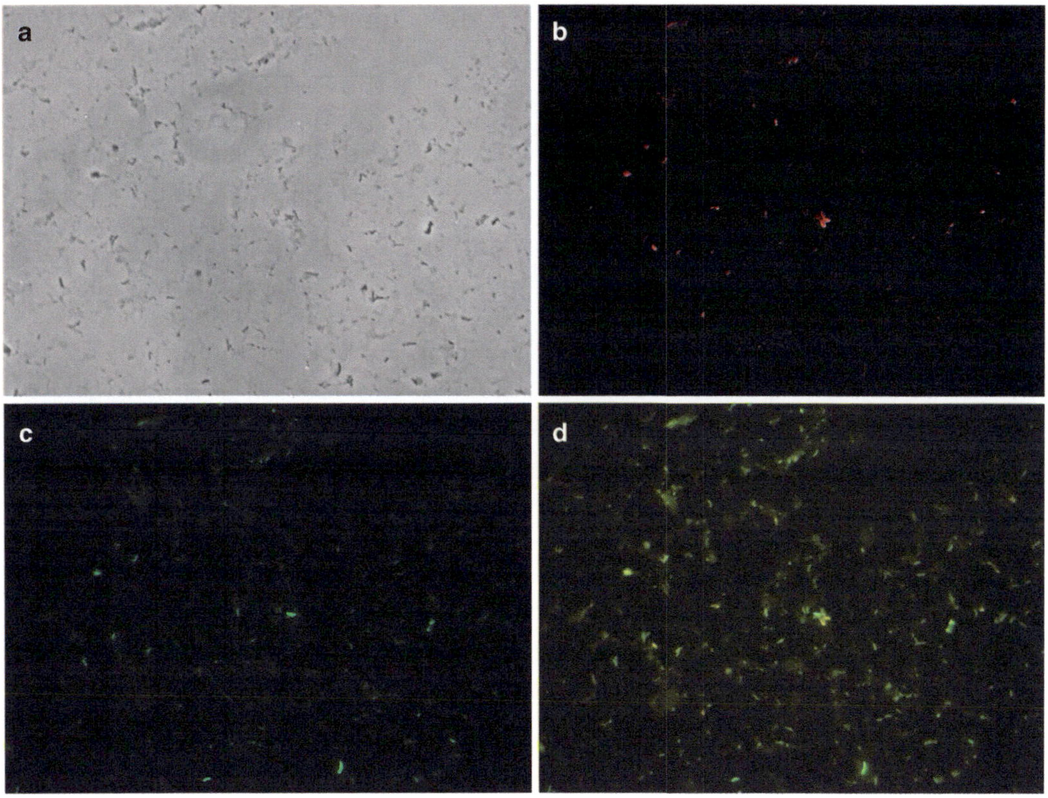

Fig. 2.2 Photomicrographs of peri-implantitis-associated submucosal biofilms. Phase-contrast observation of the sample is shown in (**a**). The sample was processed for observation by fluorescence in situ hybridization (FISH) using 16S rRNA-oligonucleotide probes labeled Cy3 for oral Spirochaetes and 6-FAM (6-fluorescein amidite) for oral Synergistetes. Epifluorescence observations show Spirochaetes in (**b**), Synergistetes in **c** and merged signals in (**d**). (Source: Belibasakis et al. [52]. Reproduced with permission from Springer Nature under the license number 4984180931936)

from reports showing that peri-implant infections may occasionally be dominated by pathogens most commonly isolated from implanted medical devices, these included *Peptostreptococcus* spp. or *Staphylococcus epidermidis* and *S. aureus* [57, 76–78]. Although these approaches permitted a faster and taxonomically more accurate identification of peri-implant communities than culture methods, they are also undermined by inherent limitations. The requirement of preselecting sets of primers and probes may skew microbial identification toward pre-targeted species, often derived from previous knowledge of periodontal communities. In this regard, closed-ended approaches may introduce a "selection" bias, which technically precludes the detection of less studied or 'unexpected' microbiota.

2.9 Profiling of Microbial Communities by Sequencing the 16s rRNA Gene

In contrast to closed-ended methods, sequencing of housekeeping genes, such as the 16S ribosomal RNA (rRNA) gene, enables microbial identification without the need of preselecting target species [79]. The 16S rRNA gene exhibits several characteristics that render it advantageous for bacterial identification and taxonomic classification. Ubiquitous in bacteria, the gene bears a series of slow-evolving over time regions (i.e., "conserved"), which sequence may be employed to recognize virtually all bacteria in a sample, intercalated with nine fast-evolving regions (variable), which sequence is taxa-specific and enables inference of taxonomic identity [80]. In other words, as these regions evolve at different rates, comparison of their sequences with reference databases enables to define the taxonomy of both ancient lineages, such as Phyla or Classes, and more recent lineages, such as Genera or Species [81].

In the late 1980s, Pace and co-workers were among the first to apply Sanger sequencing to the 16S rRNA gene to identify bacterial members from mixed consortium communities [82]. Intrinsic limitations of Sanger sequencing, however, rapidly limited the taxonomic resolution of this approach. It is costly, time-consuming, and above all, only permits a low coverage depth (low number of sequence reads) [83]. The resulting bacterial identification is therefore restricted to the predominant members of a community and omits a plethora of less represented taxa [84]. More recently, 16S based profiling of microbial communities is achieved by next-generation sequencing (NGS), that is, high-throughput DNA sequencing technologies. NGS technologies, such as formerly pyrosequencing now superseded by Illumina [85], generate thousands of sequencing reads (~5000–50,000 per sample) and have thereby led to a step change improvement in the coverage depth of analyses [86]. One particularity of the reads produced by Illumina technologies is their relatively short length (~400 bp paired-reads on MiSeq) so that only selected segments of the 16S can be analyzed. Typically, amplicons that span the variable regions V1–V2, V3–V4, or V4 alone are sequenced. Although short, clustering and alignment of these sequences on reference databases generates taxonomic profiles that confidently reach the genus level [87]. NGS of the 16S has permitted a comprehensive, system-level view of complex microbial communities (community profiling) [88, 89].

2.10 Community Profiling Reveals a Distinct Microbiota in the Peri-Implant Niche

The advent of NGS-based community profiling has unveiled an extensive bacterial diversity in the peri-implant niche and has spurred efforts to characterize peri-implant microbial communities. Compiled findings from these investigations, pioneered by Kumar and co-workers, reproducibly indicate that peri-implant sites harbor a differentially abundant microbiota and display lower microbial diversity than periodontal sites, in both health and disease [90–94]. Specifically, significant compositional differences between subgingival and submucosal microbiota were detected between healthy peri-implant and periodontal sites, as well as between peri-implantitis and periodontitis sites [90–92]. Worth mentioning here, these affections remain endogenous, polymicrobial opportunistic infections, and are therefore triggered by mixed bacterial consortia part of the "normal" oral microbiota that have undergone compositional shifts. As such, it is not the mere presence of specific bacterial taxa that distinguish peri-implant and periodontal conditions, which would imply a causal relationship. Instead, microbiota differences are reflected in taxonomic shifts toward enriched abundances of pathogenic taxa, which interplay causes the disease. That said, the presence of some allochthonous species of staphylococci in the peri-implant microbiota may constitute an exception (see next section of this chapter). Figure 2.3 provides a comparative overview of the differentially abundant taxa detected in peri-implant health and disease or periodontitis. Core taxa that were

Fig. 2.3 Schematic representation of the distinct and core microbiota associated with peri-implantitis. The Venn diagrams attempt a summative qualitative illustration of the bacterial taxa identified in the microbiota from healthy peri-implant, peri-implantitis, and periodontitis sites. Only taxa reportedly identified as significantly enriched in each condition are represented. Bacterial taxa are reported at the genus level or lower. The font size is commensurate with the frequency of identification among publications. (**a**) The microbiota from periodontitis and peri-implantitis sites are illustrated based on Kumar et al. 2012, Dabdoub et al. 2013, Maruyama et al. 2014, and Yu et al. 2019. (**b**) The microbiota from healthy implants and peri-implantitis sites are illustrated based on Kumar et al. 2012, Sanz-Martin et al. 2017, Tsigarida et al. 2015, Yu et al. 2019 and Zheng et al. 2015. Of note, bioinformatic analysis parameters, criteria of taxonomic identification, and statistical significance may vary among studies. (Source: Belibasakis et al. [4]. Adapted here in agreement with the terms of a Creative Commons CC-BY license with SAGE publishing)

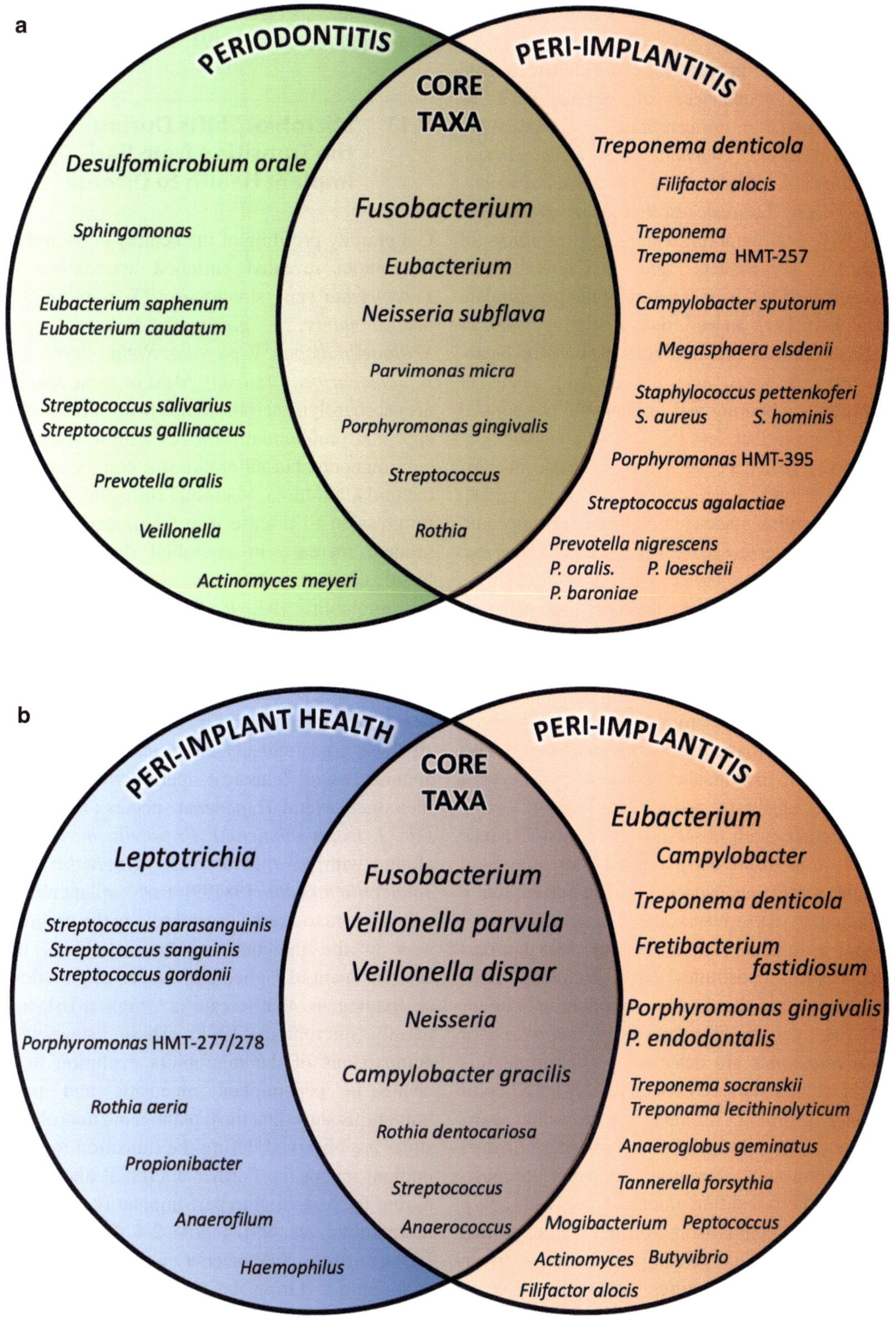
a
PERIODONTITIS
PERI-IMPLANTITIS
CORE TAXA
Desulfomicrobium orale
Sphingomonas
Eubacterium saphenum
Eubacterium caudatum
Streptococcus salivarius
Streptococcus gallinaceus
Prevotella oralis
Veillonella
Actinomyces meyeri
Fusobacterium
Eubacterium
Neisseria subflava
Parvimonas micra
Porphyromonas gingivalis
Streptococcus
Rothia
Treponema denticola
Filifactor alocis
Treponema
Treponema HMT-257
Campylobacter sputorum
Megasphaera elsdenii
Staphylococcus pettenkoferi
S. aureus S. hominis
Porphyromonas HMT-395
Streptococcus agalactiae
Prevotella nigrescens
P. oralis. P. loescheii
P. baroniae
b
PERI-IMPLANT HEALTH
PERI-IMPLANTITIS
CORE TAXA
Leptotrichia
Streptococcus parasanguinis
Streptococcus sanguinis
Streptococcus gordonii
Porphyromonas HMT-277/278
Rothia aeria
Propionibacter
Anaerofilum
Haemophilus
Fusobacterium
Veillonella parvula
Veillonella dispar
Neisseria
Campylobacter gracilis
Rothia dentocariosa
Streptococcus
Anaerococcus
Eubacterium
Campylobacter
Treponema denticola
Fretibacterium fastidiosum
Porphyromonas gingivalis
P. endodontalis
Treponema socranskii
Treponama lecithinolyticum
Anaeroglobus geminatus
Tannerella forsythia
Mogibacterium Peptococcus
Actinomyces Butyvibrio
Filifactor alocis

concomitant to these conditions are also displayed.

Overall, peri-implant sites were characterized by higher abundances of genera such as *Eubacterium*, *Anaerofilum*, *Prevotella*, *Porphyromonas*, *Selenomonas*, *Streptococcus*, *Actinomyces*, *Leptotrichia*, *Propionibacterium*, *Peptococcus*, *Lactococcus*, *Rothia*, and *Treponema* [90–94]. Furthermore, community profiling of adjacent peri-implant and periodontal sites strengthened the distinct nature of the peri-implant ecosystem [91]. Indeed, data stemming from 81 patients showed that more than 50% of the bacterial taxa detected were differentially abundant between neighboring peri-implant and periodontal sites. Even further, less than 8% of abundant species were shared between pairs of adjacent peri-implant and periodontal crevices [91]. Peri-implantitis associated communities appeared to harbor higher levels of genera such as *Treponema*, *Filifactor*, *Porphyromonas*, *Prevotella*, *Tannerella*, *Campylobacter*, or *Staphylococcus* spp., whereas *Desulfomicrobium orale*, *Sphingomonas*, *Veillonella*, *Actinomyces* spp., and non-mutans streptococci were enriched in periodontitis [91–95]. Of note, these microbiota differences between the peri-implant and periodontal niches were also observed in individuals with a past history of chronic or aggressive periodontitis [93, 94].

Together, such observations come to nuance conclusions from early reports that suggested neighboring teeth, especially those periodontally affected, to act as reservoirs of periodontopathogens for implants [96]. It remains clear that past periodontitis constitutes a risk factor for peri-implantitis and that known periodontopathogens of the genera *Treponema*, *Tannerella*, or *Porphyromonas* are detected in peri-implantitis pockets. Nonetheless, collective 16S-based community profiling strongly supports that peri-implant and periodontal sites behave as distinct ecosystems that differentially shape the composition of their residing microbiota [91–94, 97]. Taxonomic comparisons further indicate that colonization of the peri-implant niche is driven by local ecological features, rather than the proximity of nearby niches, thus extending the concept of "site-specialist" oral communities to the peri-implant ecosystem [91, 93, 94].

2.11 Microbial Shifts During the Transition from Peri-Implant Health to Disease

Community profiling of the healthy peri-implant microbiota revealed enriched abundances of *Leptotrichia* spp., streptococci (*S. sanguinis*, *S. parasanguinis*, *S. gordonii*), *Neisseria* spp., *Veillonella dispar*, *V. parvula*, *Rothia aeria*, and *R. dentocariosa* [98–100]. Most of these species are saccharolytic aerobes, aside from *Leptotrichia* spp. that preferentially thrives within anaerobic environments, but all are known commensals of the oral microbiota. Microbial shifts that underlie progression to disease were characterized by a gradual increase in microbial diversity from health to peri-implant mucositis and further to peri-implantitis [93, 98, 99]. Specifically, progression to peri-implant mucositis followed a primary ecological succession, during which newly acquired species combined with preexisting pioneer communities [98, 99]. This increased diversity was taxonomically characterized by higher abundances of "classical" periodontopathogens including several *Treponema* species (*T. socranskii*, *T. lecithinolyticum*), *Prevotella intermedia* along with *Porphyromonas gingivalis* and *Tannerella forsythia* [98, 99]. Peri-implant mucositis appears to exert a pivotal role in the progression of the infection, in that it allows the establishment of higher abundances of periodontal pathogens that create a "high-at-risk-for-harm" microbiota [99]. These stage-wise comparisons of the microbiota evolution from health to peri-implant mucositis and peri-implantitis show that most pathogenic microbiota shifts are observed during the transition to peri-implant mucositis. Further microbial alterations during the transition to peri-implantitis appeared more subtle [98, 99]. Figure 2.4 illustrates the increasing microbial diversity within submucosal communities during the typical course of peri-implant infections.

Intriguingly, one study that investigated the effects of tobacco smoking on these transitions reported that microbial shifts followed divergent pathways in smokers [99]. At healthy peri-implant sites, smokers exhibited lower microbial diversity than nonsmokers and already presented an enrichment of known periodontopathogens. The transition to peri-implant mucositis in smokers was accompanied by loss of commensals species, resulting in decreased microbial diversity, further contrasting with nonsmokers.

During the transition to peri-implantitis, the typical periodontopathogens established at the peri-implant mucositis stage were shown to persist. Several other bacterial taxa were additionally identified as enriched in peri-implantitis lesions. Typically, several other *Treponema* species that include *T. denticola, T. maltophilum* [91, 98–100], or the as-yet-uncultivated *Treponema* HMT-257 [92] were detected in higher abundance in peri-implantitis sites and correlated in some cases with radiographic bone loss, PPD, and suppuration [92]. Taxonomic characterization via 16S approaches also enabled the identification of emerging putative pathogens such as *Anaeroglobus geminatus*, *Filifactor alocis*, *Mogibacterium* spp., *Fretibacterium fastidiosum* and *Fretibacterium* HMT 360, *Desulfobulbus* HMT 041, uncharacterized taxa of *Peptostreptococcaceae* and multiple species of *Eubacterium* [93, 98, 100].

Several NGS studies also confirmed the presence of *Staphylococcus* species in significantly higher abundances in peri-implantitis communities, these mostly included *S. pettenkoferi*, *S. hominis,* and *S. aureus* [91, 93, 99]. Although staphylococci have been isolated from infective para-oral conditions such as angular cheilitis or

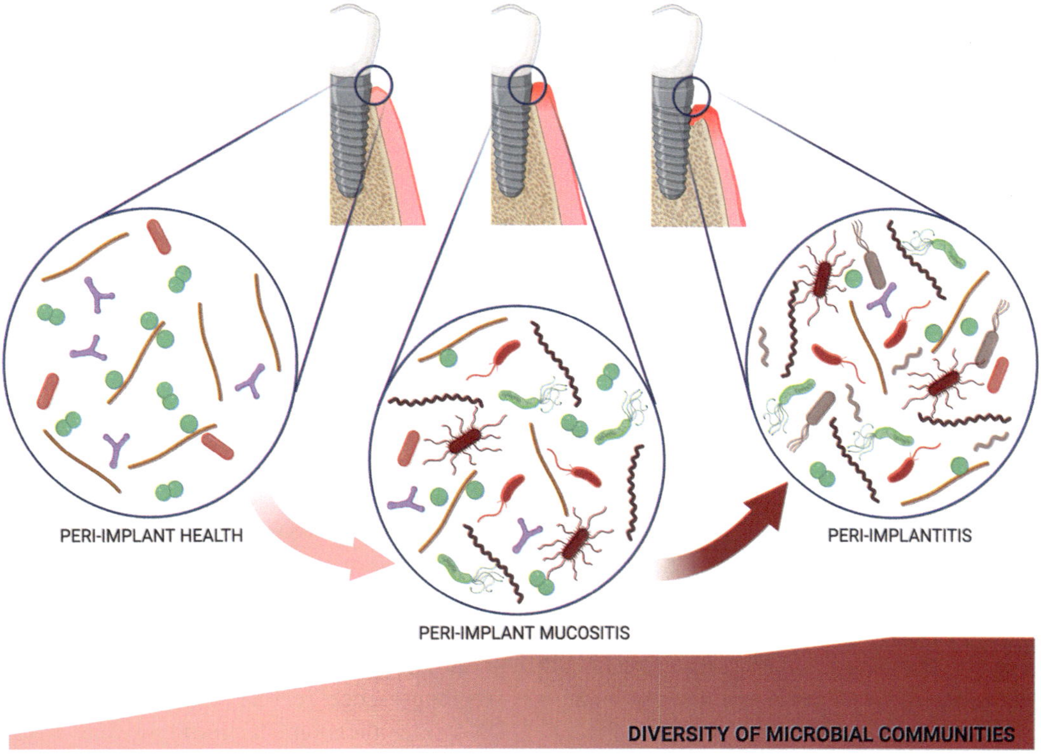

Fig. 2.4 Diversity of submucosal microbial communities during the course of peri-implant infections. The scheme illustrates the increase in microbial diversity observed during the transition from peri-implant health to peri-implant mucositis, and ultimately to peri-implantitis. (Source: the figure was initially designed using the web interface BioRender.com and published in Belibasakis et al. [4]. Reproduced in agreement with the terms of a Creative Commons CC-BY license with SAGE publishing)

parotitis, they are considered non-oral, allochthonous species, which presence in the healthy oral cavity is likely transient and originates from food or contamination from epidermal surfaces [101, 102]. However, their apparent ability to colonize artificial intra-oral surfaces, such as dentures or implants has been previously reported and attracted considerable interest [77, 103]. Staphylococci, *S. aureus* most particularly, are versatile human pathogens and leading causes of orthopedic implants infections and associated osteomyelitis. Typical virulence factors include their wide range of adhesins from the family of MSCRAMMs (Microbial Surface Components Recognizing Adhesive Matrix Molecules) [104]. These adhesins enable staphylococci to adhere to a variety of surfaces and initiate biofilm formation, which may owe an element of explanation to their increased abundances in peri-implantitis sites.

2.12 Beyond Microbial Taxonomy: Functional Profiling of Peri-Implant Communities

Whereas 16S-based approaches have undeniably led to a quantum leap in the taxonomic characterization of microbial communities associated with peri-implantitis, it is worth acknowledging some of their limitations. Most common NGS technologies to date, such as Illumina, rely on short reads that entail a selection of the variable regions to be sequenced as the entire length of the 16S cannot be considered. This feature has a twofold impact on further taxonomic assignment. First, because variable regions display unequal abilities to distinguish between bacterial taxa, the choice of specific regions may tend to over- or underestimate certain phylotypes [80, 86]. Second, because taxonomy is inferred from partial 16S sequences, the resulting taxonomic resolution is limited to the genus level, and may sometimes be stretched to the species level in the oral microbiome thanks to dedicated and well-characterized databases, such as HOMD [81, 105]. Although recent advances in long-read technologies are expected to optimize the yield of 16S approaches by enabling the full length sequencing of the gene [106, 107], more finite differences between peri-implant microbiota in health and disease likely reside at the strain level, which remains inaccessible by 16S analyses alone. More importantly, various strains of the same species may bear significantly different genomic characteristics, that is, the accessory genome, endowing them with virulence traits unique to subsets of strains [108, 109]. This is relevant because peri-implant disease is ultimately caused by the pathogenic activity of microbial communities, rather than by the mere presence of certain phylotypes.

Insights into strain-level differences may stem from shotgun metagenomic sequencing that has the potential to reassemble near-full-length metagenomes, and thereby to also inform on the functional potential (genes present transcribed or not) of these communities [110, 111]. The differential expression of virulence factors that potentiate the pathogenicity of the entire community may be assessed by metatranscriptomic approaches [112].

However, investigations aiming to elucidate functional aspects within peri-implant communities remain scarce and essentially stem from a single group and a single study cohort thus far. Specifically, Shiba et al. compared the functional profiles of peri-implantitis and periodontitis microbiota from a cohort of 12 subjects using a genome-wide metatranscriptome (RNA-seq) [113]. In this approach, total RNA is extracted from microbial communities and reverse-transcribed to a complementary DNA library to be sequenced. A near-full-length 16S rRNA sequence library was first reconstructed to simultaneously enable the taxonomic identification of bacterial communities. As this 16S library originates from transcribed RNA, it is representative of the transcriptionally active phyla, rather than of the sole presence of the gene as in traditional 16S approaches relying solely on microbial DNA identification. Interestingly, the RNA-based 16S library revealed a differentially abundant "active" microbiota between peri-implantitis and periodontitis [113]. These observations somewhat support the idea that different microbial functional profiles may underpin periodontitis and peri-implantitis diseases. Furthermore, species such as *Eubacterium nodatum*, *Peptostreptococcus stomatis,* and *Prevotella denticola* were shown to be significantly more active in peri-implantitis than periodontitis, as evidenced by RNA/DNA ratios, stemming from metatranscriptomic and metagenomic comparisons [114]. These findings are in line with previous 16S reports that also identified these taxa as significantly enriched in peri-implantitis and part of co-occurrence networks [90, 93, 100]. Further function-based assignment of mRNA sequences revealed distinct virulence profiles between healthy sites and peri-implantitis, although no specific virulence genes could be imputed to peri-implantitis. Also, mRNA-based interaction networks appeared more complex in peri-implantitis than in periodontitis, and were characterized by significant associations between species of the "red complex"; *P. gingivalis, T. forsythia,* and *T. denticola* [113].

Whereas these investigations were not devoid of limitations (small cohort size or comparisons made between meta-transcriptomic and -genomic data using different samples), these findings complement and extend previous taxonomic reports. Together, these metatranscriptomic and metagenomic data seem to illustrate that different functional profiles underlie the pathogenicity of communities found in peri-implantitis or periodontitis. Hence, functional profiling appears particularly important for a deeper understanding of the pathogenicity of a microbial community, beyond its taxonomical composition.

2.13 Summary and Conclusion

The oral cavity represents a unique ecosystem that harbors a remarkably diverse microbiota. This ecosystem is characterized by a multiplicity of ecological niches and a constant salivary flow that coats all surfaces with a proteinic pellicle. To survive in this ecosystem, oral bacteria have evolved to recognize molecular patterns of the salivary pellicle, adhere onto surfaces and generate biofilms. Within biofilms, oral bacteria coaggregate with ecologically relevant partners, exchange genetic material, communicate and establish mutually beneficial networks.

Upon insertion, dental implants offer a pristine surface, rapidly coated with a pellicle and ready to serve as a substrate for bacterial colonization and biofilm growth, similarly to natural teeth. Uncontrolled, biofilm growth will induce an inflammatory response in the peri-implant submucosa, that will alter the ecological conditions of peri-implant niche and that, in turn, will promote the proliferation of pathogenic/"inflammagenic" species. These events trigger a self-feeding vicious cycle that enhances peri-implant inflammation and may lead to the destruction of the implant-supporting tissues.

Early work that attempted to characterize the microbial communities that underpin the etiology of peri-implantitis mostly pointed to similarities with periodontitis and known periodontopathogens. The advent of NGS technologies, notably applied to the 16S rRNA gene, has considerably expanded our appreciation of the peri-implant microbiota. Indeed, compiled findings from community profiling consistently support the concept of peri-implant sites as distinct ecological niches, characterized by lower diversity than periodontal sites and by a compositionally distinct microbiota, both in health and disease. Microbial shifts during inflammatory peri-implant transitions were shown to follow a primary ecological succession characterized by the establishment of known periodontopathogens, such as representatives of the "red complex," as well as emerging putative pathogens that include *Anaeroglobus geminatus, Filifactor alocis, Eubacterium nodatum,* or *Fretibacterium fastidiosum.* Peri-implantitis-associated communities were also frequently shown to encompass allochthonous species of staphylococci.

Whereas current knowledge is somewhat limited to the taxonomic characterization of microbial communities, it is expected that more finite specificities of the peri-implant microbiota may stem from the analysis of strain-level functional characteristics. Preliminary metagenomic and metatranscriptomic data suggest indeed that differential functional profiles may underpin the etiology of peri-implantitis and periodontitis. Considering the lack of a unique therapeutic armament to tackle peri-implant infections, the identification of potential biomarker strains, or altered transcriptional profiles, may ultimately provide the basis for early detection and prevention strategies or contribute to selecting specific antimicrobial approaches.

References

1. Le Guehennec L, Soueidan A, Layrolle P, Amouriq Y. Surface treatments of titanium dental implants for rapid osseointegration. Dent Mater. 2007;23(7):844–54.
2. Salvi GE, Cosgarea R, Sculean A. Prevalence and mechanisms of peri-implant diseases. J Dent Res. 2017;96(1):31–7.
3. Belibasakis GN. Microbiological and immunopathological aspects of peri-implant diseases. Arch Oral Biol. 2014;59(1):66–72.
4. Belibasakis GN, Manoil D. Microbial community-driven etiopathogenesis of peri-implantitis. J Dent Res. 2021;100(1):21–8.
5. Heitz-Mayfield LJ, Teles R, Lang NP. Peri-implant infections. In: Lang NP, Lindhe J, editors. Clinical periodontology and implant dentistry. 6th ed. Wiley Blackwell; 2015. p. 222–37.
6. Berglundh T, Armitage G, Araujo MG, Avila-Ortiz G, Blanco J, Camargo PM, et al. Peri-implant diseases and conditions: consensus report of workgroup 4 of the 2017 world workshop on the classification of periodontal and peri-implant diseases and conditions. J Clin Periodontol. 2018;45(Suppl 20):S286–S91.
7. Hashim D, Cionca N, Combescure C, Mombelli A. The diagnosis of peri-implantitis: a systematic review on the predictive value of bleeding on probing. Clin Oral Implants Res. 2018;29(Suppl 16):276–93.
8. Ramanauskaite A, Becker K, Schwarz F. Clinical characteristics of peri-implant mucositis and peri-implantitis. Clin Oral Implants Res. 2018;29(6):551–6.
9. Rakic M, Monje A, Radovanovic S, Petkovic-Curcin A, Vojvodic D, Tatic Z. Is the personalized approach the key to improve clinical diagnosis of peri-implant conditions? The role of bone markers. J Periodontol. 2019;
10. Zitzmann NU, Berglundh T. Definition and prevalence of peri-implant diseases. J Clin Periodontol. 2008;35(8 Suppl):286–91.
11. Derks J, Tomasi C. Peri-implant health and disease. A systematic review of current epidemiology. J Clin Periodontol. 2015;42(Suppl 16):S158–71.
12. Kordbacheh Changi K, Finkelstein J, Papapanou PN. Peri-implantitis prevalence, incidence rate, and risk factors: a study of electronic health records at a U.S. dental school. Clin Oral Implants Res. 2019;30(4):306–14.
13. Kumar PS. Systemic risk factors for the development of periimplant diseases. Implant Dent. 2019;28(2):115–9.
14. Roccuzzo M, De Angelis N, Bonino L, Aglietta M. Ten-year results of a three-arm prospective cohort study on implants in periodontally compromised patients. Part 1: implant loss and radiographic bone loss. Clin Oral Implants Res. 2010;21(5):490–6.
15. Heitz-Mayfield LJ. Peri-implant diseases: diagnosis and risk indicators. J Clin Periodontol. 2008;35(8 Suppl):292–304.
16. Mombelli A, Muller N, Cionca N. The epidemiology of peri-implantitis. Clin Oral Implants Res. 2012;23(Suppl 6):67–76.
17. Lindhe J, Meyle J, Group DoEWoP. Peri-implant diseases: consensus report of the sixth european workshop on periodontology. J Clin Periodontol. 2008;35(8 Suppl):282–5.
18. Veerman EC, van den Keybus PA, Vissink A, Nieuw Amerongen AV. Human glandular salivas: their separate collection and analysis. Eur J Oral Sci. 1996;104(4 (Pt 1)):346–52.
19. Siqueira WL, Salih E, Wan DL, Helmerhorst EJ, Oppenheim FG. Proteome of human minor salivary gland secretion. J Dent Res. 2008;87(5):445–50.
20. Hall MW, Singh N, Ng KF, Lam DK, Goldberg MB, Tenenbaum HC, et al. Inter-personal diversity and temporal dynamics of dental, tongue, and salivary microbiota in the healthy oral cavity. NPJ Biofilms Microbiomes. 2017;3:2.
21. Bostanci N, Belibasakis GN. Gingival crevicular fluid and its immune mediators in the proteomic era. Periodontol 2000. 2018;76(1):68–84.
22. Proctor DM, Relman DA. The landscape ecology and microbiota of the human nose, mouth, and throat. Cell Host Microbe. 2017;21(4):421–32.
23. Avila M, Ojcius DM, Yilmaz O. The oral microbiota: living with a permanent guest. DNA Cell Biol. 2009;28(8):405–11.
24. Costalonga M, Herzberg MC. The oral microbiome and the immunobiology of periodontal disease and caries. Immunol Lett. 2014;162(2 Pt A):22–38.
25. Dewhirst FE, Chen T, Izard J, Paster BJ, Tanner AC, Yu WH, et al. The human oral microbiome. J Bacteriol. 2010;192(19):5002–17.
26. Proctor DM, Shelef KM, Gonzalez A, Davis CL, Dethlefsen L, Burns AR, et al. Microbial biogeography and ecology of the mouth and implications for periodontal diseases. Periodontol 2000. 2020;82(1):26–41.
27. Mark Welch JL, Rossetti BJ, Rieken CW, Dewhirst FE, Borisy GG. Biogeography of a human oral microbiome at the micron scale. Proc Natl Acad Sci USA. 2016;113(6):E791–800.

28. Mark Welch JL, Dewhirst FE, Borisy GG. Biogeography of the oral microbiome: the site-specialist hypothesis. Annu Rev Microbiol. 2019;73:335–58.
29. Roberts FA, Darveau RP. Microbial protection and virulence in periodontal tissue as a function of polymicrobial communities: symbiosis and dysbiosis. Periodontol. 2015;69(1):18–27.
30. Stewart PS, Franklin MJ. Physiological heterogeneity in biofilms. Nat Rev Microbiol. 2008;6(3):199–210.
31. Kolenbrander PE, Palmer RJ Jr, Periasamy S, Jakubovics NS. Oral multispecies biofilm development and the key role of cell-cell distance. Nat Rev Microbiol. 2010;8(7):471–80.
32. Siqueira WL, Custodio W, McDonald EE. New insights into the composition and functions of the acquired enamel pellicle. J Dent Res. 2012;91(12):1110–8.
33. Jensen JL, Lamkin MS, Oppenheim FG. Adsorption of human salivary proteins to hydroxyapatite: a comparison between whole saliva and glandular salivary secretions. J Dent Res. 1992;71(9):1569–76.
34. Li J, Helmerhorst EJ, Leone CW, Troxler RF, Yaskell T, Haffajee AD, et al. Identification of early microbial colonizers in human dental biofilm. J Appl Microbiol. 2004;97(6):1311–8.
35. Kaplan CW, Lux R, Haake SK, Shi W. The Fusobacterium nucleatum outer membrane protein RadD is an arginine-inhibitable adhesin required for inter-species adherence and the structured architecture of multispecies biofilm. Mol Microbiol. 2009;71(1):35–47.
36. Hoare A, Wang H, Meethil A, Abusleme L, Hong BY, Moutsopoulos NM, et al. A cross-species interaction with a symbiotic commensal enables cell-density-dependent growth and in vivo virulence of an oral pathogen. ISME J. 2020;
37. Diaz PI, Chalmers NI, Rickard AH, Kong C, Milburn CL, Palmer RJ Jr, et al. Molecular characterization of subject-specific oral microflora during initial colonization of enamel. Appl Environ Microbiol. 2006;72(4):2837–48.
38. Dige I, Raarup MK, Nyengaard JR, Kilian M, Nyvad B. Actinomyces naeslundii in initial dental biofilm formation. Microbiology (Reading). 2009;155(Pt 7):2116–26.
39. Marsh PD, Zaura E. Dental biofilm: ecological interactions in health and disease. J Clin Periodontol. 2017;44(Suppl 18):S12–22.
40. Bolstad AI, Jensen HB, Bakken V. Taxonomy, biology, and periodontal aspects of Fusobacterium nucleatum. Clin Microbiol Rev. 1996;9(1):55–71.
41. Bradshaw DJ, Homer KA, Marsh PD, Beighton D. Metabolic cooperation in oral microbial communities during growth on mucin. Microbiology (Reading). 1994;140(Pt 12):3407–12.
42. Burmolle M, Ren D, Bjarnsholt T, Sorensen SJ. Interactions in multispecies biofilms: do they actually matter? Trends Microbiol. 2014;22(2):84–91.
43. Parsek MR, Greenberg EP. Sociomicrobiology: the connections between quorum sensing and biofilms. Trends Microbiol. 2005;13(1):27–33.
44. Abisado RG, Benomar S, Klaus JR, Dandekar AA, Chandler JR. Bacterial quorum wensing and microbial community interactions. mBio. 2018;9(3)
45. Fuqua C, Greenberg EP. Listening in on bacteria: acyl-homoserine lactone signalling. Nat Rev Mol Cell Biol. 2002;3(9):685–95.
46. Rickard AH, Palmer RJ Jr, Blehert DS, Campagna SR, Semmelhack MF, Egland PG, et al. Autoinducer 2: a concentration-dependent signal for mutualistic bacterial biofilm growth. Mol Microbiol. 2006;60(6):1446–56.
47. Frias J, Olle E, Alsina M. Periodontal pathogens produce quorum sensing signal molecules. Infect Immun. 2001;69(5):3431–4.
48. Kolenbrander PE, Andersen RN, Blehert DS, Egland PG, Foster JS, Palmer RJ Jr. Communication among oral bacteria. Microbiol Mol Biol Rev. 2002;66(3):486–505. table of contents
49. Heitz-Mayfield LJ, Lang NP. Comparative biology of chronic and aggressive periodontitis vs. peri-implantitis. Periodontol. 2010;53:167–81.
50. Lindhe J, Karring T, Araujo M. Anatomy of periodontal tissues. In: Lang NP, Lindhe J, editors. Clinical periodontology and implant dentistry. 6th ed. Wiley Blackwell; 2015. p. 3–47.
51. Lindhe J, Wennström JL, Berglundh T. The mucosa at teeth and implants. In: Lang NP, Lindhe J, editors. Clinical periodontology and implant dentistry. 6th ed. Wiley Blackwell; 2015. p. 83–99.
52. Belibasakis GN, Charalampakis G, Bostanci N, Stadlinger B. Peri-implant infections of oral biofilm etiology. Adv Exp Med Biol. 2015;830:69–84.
53. Edgerton M, Lo SE, Scannapieco FA. Experimental salivary pellicles formed on titanium surfaces mediate adhesion of streptococci. Int J Oral Maxillofac Implants. 1996;11(4):443–9.
54. Quirynen M, Vogels R, Pauwels M, Haffajee AD, Socransky SS, Uzel NG, et al. Initial subgingival colonization of 'pristine' pockets. J Dent Res. 2005;84(4):340–4.
55. Leonhardt A, Olsson J, Dahlen G. Bacterial colonization on titanium, hydroxyapatite, and amalgam surfaces in vivo. J Dent Res. 1995;74(9):1607–12.
56. Frojd V, Linderback P, Wennerberg A, Chavez de Paz L, Svensater G, Davies JR. Effect of nanoporous TiO2 coating and anodized Ca2+ modification of titanium surfaces on early microbial biofilm formation. BMC Oral Health. 2011;11:8.
57. Furst MM, Salvi GE, Lang NP, Persson GR. Bacterial colonization immediately after installation on oral titanium implants. Clin Oral Implants Res. 2007;18(4):501–8.
58. Lang NP, Berglundh T. Working Group 4 of Seventh European Workshop on P. Periimplant diseases: where are we now?—Consensus of the Seventh European Workshop on periodontology. J Clin Periodontol. 2011;38(Suppl 11):178–81.

59. Payne JB, Johnson PG, Kok CR, Gomes-Neto JC, Ramer-Tait AE, Schmid MJ, et al. Subgingival microbiome colonization and cytokine production during early dental implant healing. mSphere. 2017;2(6)
60. Schincaglia GP, Hong BY, Rosania A, Barasz J, Thompson A, Sobue T, et al. Clinical, immune, and microbiome traits of gingivitis and peri-implant mucositis. J Dent Res. 2017;96(1):47–55.
61. Kumar PS, Leys EJ, Bryk JM, Martinez FJ, Moeschberger ML, Griffen AL. Changes in periodontal health status are associated with bacterial community shifts as assessed by quantitative 16S cloning and sequencing. J Clin Microbiol. 2006;44(10):3665–73.
62. Hajishengallis G, Darveau RP, Curtis MA. The keystone-pathogen hypothesis. Nat Rev Microbiol. 2012;10(10):717–25.
63. Lindhe J, Berglundh T, Ericsson I, Liljenberg B, Marinello C. Experimental breakdown of peri-implant and periodontal tissues. A study in the beagle dog. Clin Oral Implants Res. 1992;3(1):9–16.
64. Charalampakis G, Belibasakis GN. Microbiome of peri-implant infections: lessons from conventional, molecular and metagenomic analyses. Virulence. 2015;6(3):183–7.
65. Mombelli A, Lang NP. The diagnosis and treatment of peri-implantitis. Periodontol 2000. 1998;17:63–76.
66. Mombelli A, van Oosten MA, Schurch E Jr, Land NP. The microbiota associated with successful or failing osseointegrated titanium implants. Oral Microbiol Immunol. 1987;2(4):145–51.
67. Bower RC, Radny NR, Wall CD, Henry PJ. Clinical and microscopic findings in edentulous patients 3 years after incorporation of osseointegrated implant-supported bridgework. J Clin Periodontol. 1989;16(9):580–7.
68. Pontoriero R, Tonelli MP, Carnevale G, Mombelli A, Nyman SR, Lang NP. Experimentally induced peri-implant mucositis. A clinical study in humans. Clin Oral Implants Res. 1994;5(4):254–9.
69. Mombelli A, Decaillet F. The characteristics of biofilms in peri-implant disease. J Clin Periodontol. 2011;38(Suppl 11):203–13.
70. Devides SL, Franco AT. Evaluation of peri-implant microbiota using the polymerase chain reaction in completely edentulous patients before and after placement of implant-supported prostheses submitted to immediate load. Int J Oral Maxillofac Implants. 2006;21(2):262–9.
71. Galassi F, Kaman WE, Anssari Moin D, van der Horst J, Wismeijer D, Crielaard W, et al. Comparing culture, real-time PCR and fluorescence resonance energy transfer technology for detection of Porphyromonas gingivalis in patients with or without peri-implant infections. J Periodontal Res. 2012;47(5):616–25.
72. Al-Radha AS, Pal A, Pettemerides AP, Jenkinson HF. Molecular analysis of microbiota associated with peri-implant diseases. J Dent. 2012;40(11):989–98.
73. Hultin M, Gustafsson A, Hallstrom H, Johansson LA, Ekfeldt A, Klinge B. Microbiological findings and host response in patients with peri-implantitis. Clin Oral Implants Res. 2002;13(4):349–58.
74. Shibli JA, Melo L, Ferrari DS, Figueiredo LC, Faveri M, Feres M. Composition of supra- and subgingival biofilm of subjects with healthy and diseased implants. Clin Oral Implants Res. 2008;19(10):975–82.
75. Belibasakis GN, Mir-Mari J, Sahrmann P, Sanz-Martin I, Schmidlin PR, Jung RE. Clinical association of Spirochaetes and Synergistetes with peri-implantitis. Clin Oral Implants Res. 2016;27(6):656–61.
76. Salvi GE, Furst MM, Lang NP, Persson GR. One-year bacterial colonization patterns of Staphylococcus aureus and other bacteria at implants and adjacent teeth. Clin Oral Implants Res. 2008;19(3):242–8.
77. Persson GR, Renvert S. Cluster of bacteria associated with peri-implantitis. Clin Implant Dent Relat Res. 2014;16(6):783–93.
78. Renvert S, Lindahl C, Renvert H, Persson GR. Clinical and microbiological analysis of subjects treated with Branemark or AstraTech implants: a 7-year follow-up study. Clin Oral Implants Res. 2008;19(4):342–7.
79. Woese CR. Interpreting the universal phylogenetic tree. Proc Natl Acad Sci USA. 2000;97(15):8392–6.
80. Kuczynski J, Lauber CL, Walters WA, Parfrey LW, Clemente JC, Gevers D, et al. Experimental and analytical tools for studying the human microbiome. Nat Rev Genet. 2011;13(1):47–58.
81. Yarza P, Yilmaz P, Pruesse E, Glockner FO, Ludwig W, Schleifer KH, et al. Uniting the classification of cultured and uncultured bacteria and archaea using 16S rRNA gene sequences. Nat Rev Microbiol. 2014;12(9):635–45.
82. Olsen GJ, Lane DJ, Giovannoni SJ, Pace NR, Stahl DA. Microbial ecology and evolution: a ribosomal RNA approach. Annu Rev Microbiol. 1986;40:337–65.
83. Wang XV, Blades N, Ding J, Sultana R, Parmigiani G. Estimation of sequencing error rates in short reads. BMC Bioinformatics. 2012;13:185.
84. Kumar KR, Cowley MJ, Davis RL. Next-generation sequencing and emerging technologies. Semin Thromb Hemost. 2019;45(7):661–73.
85. Goodwin S, McPherson JD, McCombie WR. Coming of age: ten years of next-generation sequencing technologies. Nat Rev Genet. 2016;17(6):333–51.
86. Bukin YS, Galachyants YP, Morozov IV, Bukin SV, Zakharenko AS, Zemskaya TI. The effect of 16S rRNA region choice on bacterial community metabarcoding results. Sci Data. 2019;6:190007.
87. Wade WG, Prosdocimi EM. Profiling of oral bacterial communities. J Dent Res. 2020; 22034520914594
88. Rausch P, Ruhlemann M, Hermes BM, Doms S, Dagan T, Dierking K, et al. Comparative analysis of amplicon and metagenomic sequencing methods

reveals key features in the evolution of animal metaorganisms. Microbiome. 2019;7(1):133.
89. Shaiber A, Eren AM. Composite metagenome-assembled genomes reduce the quality of public genome repositories. mBio. 2019;10(3)
90. Kumar PS, Mason MR, Brooker MR, O'Brien K. Pyrosequencing reveals unique microbial signatures associated with healthy and failing dental implants. J Clin Periodontol. 2012;39(5):425–33.
91. Dabdoub SM, Tsigarida AA, Kumar PS. Patient-specific analysis of periodontal and peri-implant microbiomes. J Dent Res. 2013;92(12 Suppl):168S–75S.
92. Maruyama N, Maruyama F, Takeuchi Y, Aikawa C, Izumi Y, Nakagawa I. Intraindividual variation in core microbiota in peri-implantitis and periodontitis. Sci Rep. 2014;4:6602.
93. Sousa V, Nibali L, Spratt D, Dopico J, Mardas N, Petrie A, et al. Peri-implant and periodontal microbiome diversity in aggressive periodontitis patients: a pilot study. Clin Oral Implants Res. 2017;28(5):558–70.
94. Apatzidou D, Lappin DF, Hamilton G, Papadopoulos CA, Konstantinidis A, Riggio MP. Microbiome of peri-implantitis affected and healthy dental sites in patients with a history of chronic periodontitis. Arch Oral Biol. 2017;83:145–52.
95. Gao X, Zhou J, Sun X, Li X, Zhou Y. Diversity analysis of subgingival microbial bacteria in peri-implantitis in Uygur population. Medicine (Baltimore). 2018;97(5):e9774.
96. Papaioannou W, Quirynen M, Nys M, van Steenberghe D. The effect of periodontal parameters on the subgingival microbiota around implants. Clin Oral Implants Res. 1995;6(4):197–204.
97. Yu XL, Chan Y, Zhuang L, Lai HC, Lang NP, Keung Leung W, et al. Intra-oral single-site comparisons of periodontal and peri-implant microbiota in health and disease. Clin Oral Implants Res. 2019;30(8):760–76.
98. Zheng H, Xu L, Wang Z, Li L, Zhang J, Zhang Q, et al. Subgingival microbiome in patients with healthy and ailing dental implants. Sci Rep. 2015;5:10948.
99. Tsigarida AA, Dabdoub SM, Nagaraja HN, Kumar PS. The influence of smoking on the peri-implant microbiome. J Dent Res. 2015;94(9):1202–17.
100. Sanz-Martin I, Doolittle-Hall J, Teles RP, Patel M, Belibasakis GN, Hammerle CHF, et al. Exploring the microbiome of healthy and diseased peri-implant sites using Illumina sequencing. J Clin Periodontol. 2017;44(12):1274–84.
101. Smith AJ, Jackson MS, Bagg J. The ecology of Staphylococcus species in the oral cavity. J Med Microbiol. 2001;50(11):940–6.
102. Marsh PD, Lewis MAO, Rogers H, Williams DW, Wilson M. The mouth as a microbial habitat. In: Elsevier, editor. Oral microbiology. 6th ed. Churchill Livingstone; 2016. p. 10–25.
103. Marsh PD, Lewis MAO, Rogers H, Williams DW, Wilson M. Dental plaque. In: Elsevier, editor. Oral microbiology. 6th ed. Churchill Livingstone; 2016. p. 81–111.
104. Foster TJ. The MSCRAMM family of cell-wall-anchored surface proteins of gram-positive cocci. Trends Microbiol. 2019;27(11):927–41.
105. Chen T, Yu WH, Izard J, Baranova OV, Lakshmanan A, Dewhirst FE. The human oral microbiome database: a web accessible resource for investigating oral microbe taxonomic and genomic information. Database (Oxford). 2010; 2010:baq013
106. Callahan BJ, Wong J, Heiner C, Oh S, Theriot CM, Gulati AS, et al. High-throughput amplicon sequencing of the full-length 16S rRNA gene with single-nucleotide resolution. Nucleic Acids Res. 2019;47(18):e103.
107. Schloss PD, Jenior ML, Koumpouras CC, Westcott SL, Highlander SK. Sequencing 16S rRNA gene fragments using the PacBio SMRT DNA sequencing system. Peer J. 2016;4:e1869.
108. Baron EJ. Classification. In: Baron S, editor. Medical microbiology. Galveston (TX); 1996.
109. Quince C, Walker AW, Simpson JT, Loman NJ, Segata N. Shotgun metagenomics, from sampling to analysis. Nat Biotechnol. 2017;35(9):833–44.
110. Alcaraz LD, Belda-Ferre P, Cabrera-Rubio R, Romero H, Simon-Soro A, Pignatelli M, et al. Identifying a healthy oral microbiome through metagenomics. Clin Microbiol Infect. 2012;18(Suppl 4):54–7.
111. Bowers RM, Kyrpides NC, Stepanauskas R, Harmon-Smith M, Doud D, Reddy TBK, et al. Minimum information about a single amplified genome (MISAG) and a metagenome-assembled genome (MIMAG) of bacteria and archaea. Nat Biotechnol. 2017;35(8):725–31.
112. Sorek R, Cossart P. Prokaryotic transcriptomics: a new view on regulation, physiology and pathogenicity. Nat Rev Genet. 2010;11(1):9–16.
113. Shiba T, Watanabe T, Kachi H, Koyanagi T, Maruyama N, Murase K, et al. Distinct interacting core taxa in co-occurrence networks enable discrimination of polymicrobial oral diseases with similar symptoms. Sci Rep. 2016;6:30997.
114. Komatsu K, Shiba T, Takeuchi Y, Watanabe T, Koyanagi T, Nemoto T, et al. Discriminating microbial community structure between peri-implantitis and periodontitis with integrated metagenomic, metatranscriptomic, and network analysis. Front Cell Infect Microbiol. 2020;10:596490.

Host Immune Response to Dental Implants

3

Nagihan Bostanci, Angelika Silberiesen, Kai Bao, and Ali Gurkan

3.1 Host Defense in Dental Implant Environments

3.1.1 Osseointegration and Host Response

Biocompatibility and biostability are the key properties of dental implants in the "oral environment," in order to optimize their performance before or after functional loading. Biomaterials involving dental implants should be able to directly interact with their oral environment and adapt to the needs of the living organ [1]. Clinical biocompatibility rather refers not to a generic property of a biomaterial, but of a biomaterial-host system [2]. Uneventful host defense to dental implant insertion is not necessarily "not at all a response in the tissue"; however, it starts with more a favorable immune response that promotes wound healing around the jawbone and soft mucosal tissue.

Dental implants are placed in the jawbone through surgical procedures that create an "implant wound" in the bone and soft tissue (Fig. 3.1). Attempts to minimize wound area and surgical trauma to bone and soft tissues are crucial to ultimately reduce the response in peri-implant tissues, thus leading to a faster wound healing and a more favorable host-biomaterial interaction (Fig. 3.2). Soft tissue healing is indicated by the formation of a mucosal barrier (biological seal) at the soft tissue-transmucosal interface, while a direct structural and functional connection between the bone and the implant interface is defined as "osseointegration," or has earlier been characterized as "functional ankylosis" [3].

Bone tissue healing around dental implants includes an initial homeostasis phase, a pro-inflammatory phase, a cell proliferation phase, and a final remodeling phase [4]. In experimental animal models, the inflammatory phase is initiated as soon as 2 h following implant placement and is characterized by recruitment of leukocytes, which is followed by an increased number of fibroblasts and presence of osteoclasts in the recipient bone, starting from at 4 days to 1 week (i.e., proliferative phase) [5]. Polymorphonuclear granulocytes are the dominating leukocytes on all surfaces followed by monocytes. Stabilization of the blood clot to the implant surface and cell adhesion are important steps for successful integration and mediated through protein adsorption to the implant surface [6]. Interestingly, in humans, there is no obvious osteoclastic activity during the proliferative phase. The remodeling

N. Bostanci (✉) · A. Silberiesen · K. Bao
Section of Periodontology and Oral Health, Division of Oral Diseases, Department of Dental Medicine, Karolinska Institute, Stockholm, Sweden
e-mail: nagihan.bostanci@ki.se; angelika.silbereisen@ki.se; kai.bao@ki.se

A. Gurkan
School of Dentistry, Department of Periodontology, Ege University, Bornova, Turkey
e-mail: ali.gurkan@ege.edu.tr

P. Neelakantan, A. Princy Solomon (eds.), *Dental Implants and Oral Microbiome Dysbiosis*,
https://doi.org/10.1007/978-3-030-99014-5_3

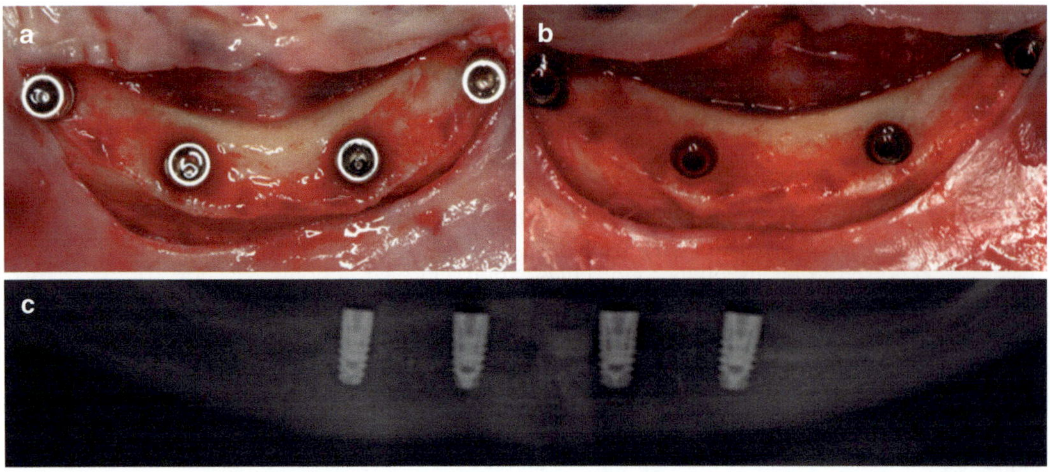

Fig. 3.1 Bone wound healing around implants. Achievement and maintenance of osseointegration and mucosal seal formation depends on establishment of a long-term equilibrium between host cells and titanium. Early and late host immune reactions to dental implant procedures are immune-inflammatory response, angiogenesis, and osteogenesis. Healing process that starts with the stabilization of the blood clot and respective occurrence of homeostasis, pro-inflammatory, cell proliferation, and finally remodeling phases eventually leads to osseointegration of the implants. (**a**) Insertion of four self-tapping implants to osteotomy sites at edentulous lower jaw; (**b**) surgical site following disconnection of transfer pieces; (**c**) radiographic images at the first-stage surgery

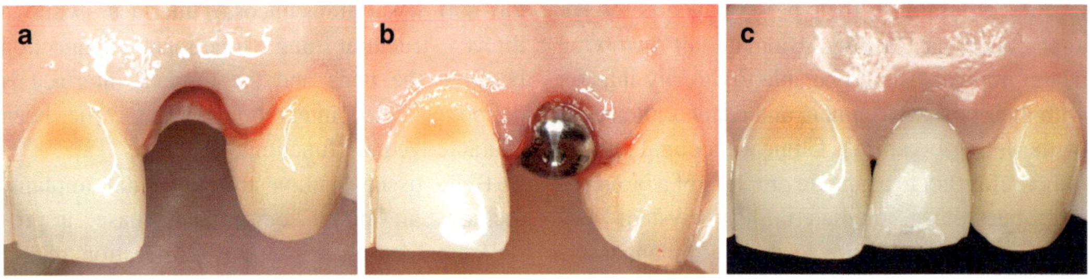

Fig. 3.2 Peri-implant soft tissue healing around healing abutments. (**a**) Edentulous space of upper left lateral incisor after 8 months of socket preservation and provisionalization; (**b**) healing abutment in place following placement of a dental implant via flapless guided surgery; (**c**) soft tissue healing around healing abutment over 3 days after immediate restoration with a temporary crown

phase begins at around 2 weeks by an increased number of osteoclasts and may extend to 12 weeks until most of the woven bone is replaced by lamellar bone. Transition to the remodeling phase in humans shows more delayed onset at least 2 weeks, compared with beagle dogs [7].

Implant wound healing in the jawbone is coordinated by structural and immune cells that interact with each other via growth factors, cytokines, chemokines, and matrix proteins [5, 8, 9]. Gene expression analysis of peri-implant tissue at early stages of tissue healing indicates that the pro-inflammatory response associated pathways are upregulated during the early stages of osseointegration around day 4. Thereafter, around day 14, these pathways are replaced with the upregulation of genes associated with osteogenesis-related mechanisms [10, 11]. Tissue-resident macrophages are an integral part of the osseointegration and wound healing process and can release several pro-inflammatory cytokines or growth factors in response to the injury caused by surgery

[12]. Multiple cytokine profiling of peri-implant crevicular fluid collected 2, 4, 8, 12, and 24 weeks following implant placement in humans showed that a vast array of cytokines peaked at week 2 after implant insertion, before decreasing at week 4 or week 8, then remaining steady at least until week 24, postoperatively [13, 14]. These findings highlighted that early weeks following implant insertion are crucial time points of successful wound healing around implants, and support the previously reported histological observations and gene expressions data.

This type of immune response during the early stages of osseointegration around implants can be considered as "sterile inflammation" that is resolved if there are no other complications. The immune response features of the bone-implant interface may be affected by several factors including implant surface characteristics/design, surgical procedure for implant bed preparation, or implant-abutment interface configuration [15]. Implant surface topography modifications may promote osteogenesis by osteoblasts, but much less is known about their potential effect on immune cell modulation and control of inflammation [16–19]. Hotchkiss and coworkers. [16] showed that macrophages cultured in vitro on implants with high surface wettability or implants with a combination of high-energy and altered surface chemistry produce an anti-inflammatory host response that reduces extended pro-inflammatory factor release. A better understanding of the effect of implant surface characteristics on a wound-healing microenvironment may enhance implant success and prevent early implant loss, which has also been postulated to be associated with a provoked foreign body reaction [20, 21]. Several other studies also reported foreign body or hypersensitivity reactions as a result of the implant material itself [22–26]. In healthy individuals with a maximum of 3 successfully restored titanium dental implants, blood levels of lactate dehydrogenase (LDH) and total protein levels were significantly higher 6 months after implant placement compared to baseline [22]. However, none of the levels were of clinical relevance. In addition, blood lymphocytes and monocytes from healthy individuals, baring or not dental implants, were isolated and their cell activity and cytokine production capacity to titanium were assessed in vitro [23]. T-cell proliferation was similar in both groups, but IL-1β, IL-6, and tumor necrosis factor (TNF)-α production was significantly lower in individuals with implants. Furthermore, several studies investigated the in vitro effect of blood on titanium and/or zirconia dental implants [24–26]. For this, unused implants were incubated in blood from a healthy donor and were harvested after 1, 8 , and 24 h to assess gene expression of IL-8 to the implant material [24, 26]. IL-8 gene expressions and IL-1β plasma protein levels were significantly increased, compared to baseline, irrespective of the implant type [24, 25].

On the other hand, dental implant coatings may wear off over time, leading to titanium corrosion and titanium particle release [27]. Berbel et al. showed that limited access to oxygen in the peri-implant defect environment reduces the resistance of implants to corrosion [28]. Although it is not clear whether such particle release can lead to a hypersensitivity reaction, there is evidence that titanium ions can induce inflammasome expression by macrophages and activate the release of pro-inflammatory cytokines [29]. This is in line with findings a greater number of macrophages containing titanium particles was found in the areas in close contact with the implant surface [30].

During wound healing following implant installation, bone modeling occurs that may result in some reduction of the marginal bone level coupled to immunological reactions. Early bone loss process can be a result of multifactorial factors, including intrinsic and extrinsic ones (Fig. 3.3). Among these, less traumatic osteotomy modalities for implant bed preparation may lead to the reduction of pro-inflammatory response at an early stage [31]. Piezoelectric surgery, a minimally invasive technique to prepare the implant bed has been shown to modify and reduce bone-destructive inflammatory molecules during implant osseointegration [13, 14, 32].

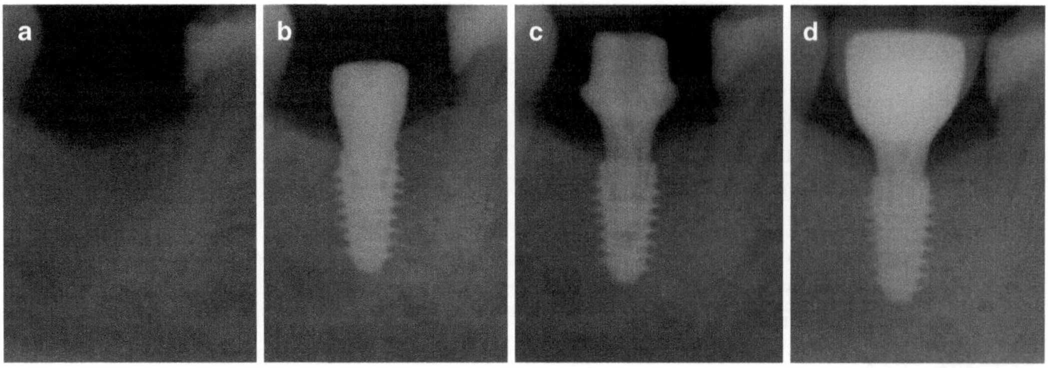

Fig. 3.3 Osseointegration and crestal bone levels around the implants. Early peri-implant crestal bone loss is a multifactorial phenomenon including several modifiable or avoidable factors related to patients, implant design, surgical and prosthetic interventions [31, 33]. Current strategies target achievement of minimal or no crestal bone loss around dental implants. (**a**) Healed lower molar extraction site; (**b**) healing abutment placed simultaneously immediately after guided flapless implant surgery; (**c**) implant was immediately restored with provisional crown and non-functionally loaded; (**d**) osseointegrated implant with definitive prosthesis. Note absence of crestal bone loss and maintenance of the successful osseointegration (Surgery Prof Ali Gurkan, Prosthetics Prof Bulent Gokce)

3.1.2 Peri-Implant Soft Tissue Integration and Host Response

The formation of a soft tissue barrier at implants is the result of a maturation process within the connective tissue and epithelial proliferation during wound healing. Peri-implant soft tissue healing is described as a "gingival seal" formation [34] (Fig. 3.4). When assessed at the microscopic level, the healthy peri-implant mucosa in humans can reach up to 3.6 mm height and consists of a 1.9 mm sulcular and junctional epithelium (keratinized and nonkeratinized) and a 1.7 mm underlying connective tissue [35]. While the apical part of peri-implant mucosa creates a connective tissue adhesion zone with limited vascularization, the coronal part consists of junctional and sulcular epithelium with some vascularity [12, 36]. Blood supply of peri-implant mucosa is provided solely by the supraperiosteal blood vessels [37]. Therefore, peri-implant mucosa may have an impaired immune response compared to gingiva around teeth [38].

Experiments in dogs and humans have documented the cellular events in the connective tissue interface portion of the peri-implant mucosa during the early stages of healing [12, 34]. Two hours after implant installation, blood coagulum was observed in the spaces between the mucosa and the implant and between the mucosa and bone. Following surgery at 4 days, there was an influx of the neutrophil granulocytes into blood cloth that degraded the coagulum and created a leukocyte-infiltrated fibrin network. It was demonstrated that macrophages were distributed in the connective tissue throughout the entire healing period. Acute inflammatory changes at week 1 were reflected as an increase in PICF volumes [38]. The PICF content showed higher expression of specific pro-inflammatory mediators in implants compared to teeth during post-operative healing, revealing a more robust response to surgical trauma in peri-implant compared to periodontal tissues [38, 39]. While T and B lymphocytes were densely packed in the connective tissue at 2 weeks of healing, then their numbers declined from 4 to 8 weeks of healing in parallel with reduced vascularity [12]. Furthermore, the first signs of epithelial proliferation were observed in specimens representing 1–2 weeks of healing and a mature junctional epithelium occurred after 6–8 weeks of healing. The collagen fibers of the mucosa were organized parallel to the implant surface after 4 or 6 weeks of healing without insertion into the implant surface. Collectively, the soft tissue attachment to implants is established after several weeks following surgery and induction and resolution of inflammation appear to be a hallmark for the healing process of the peri-implant mucosa (Fig. 3.4).

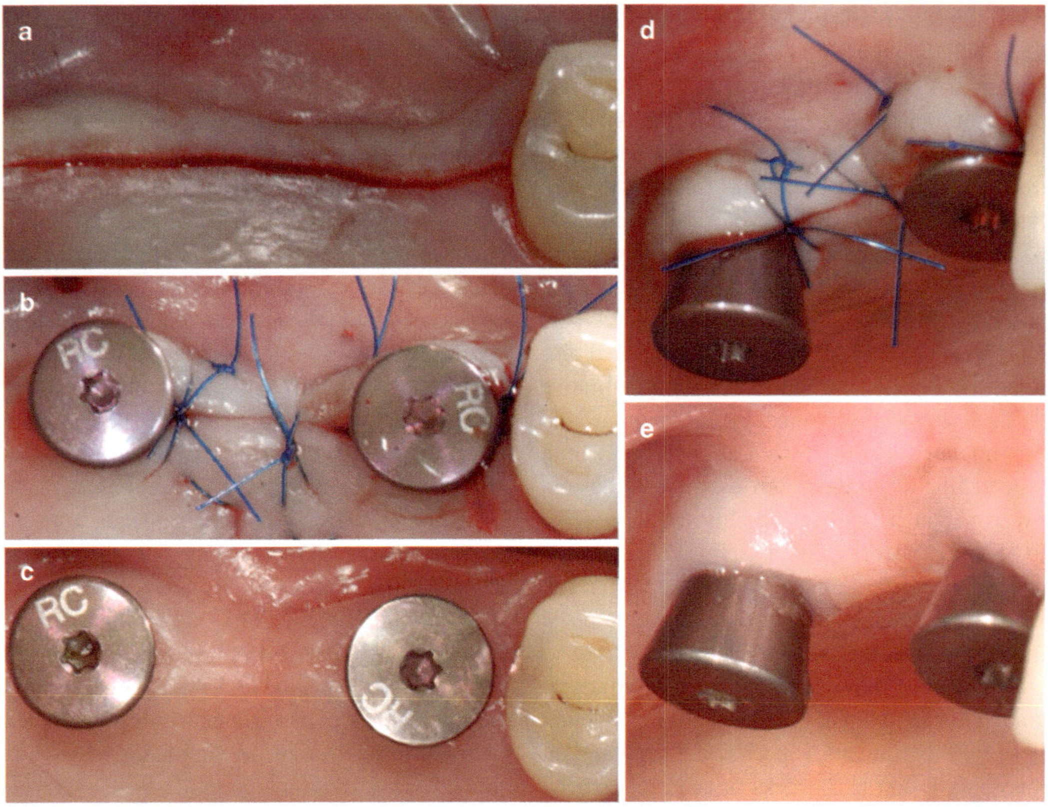

Fig. 3.4 Peri-implant soft tissue integration and host response around implants. During an uneventful wound healing period around implants, formation of a mucosal seal is characterized with proliferation of epithelium and maturation of connective tissue. The soft tissue undergoes pivotal changes including shift of the provisional matrix to a collagen fiber-dominated one and alterations in volume, cellular content, organization, and dimension and reaches its final characteristics within 6–8 weeks. (**a**) Mid-crestal incision prepared for second-stage surgery in order to uncover 2 implants left for submerged healing; (**b**) connection of healing abutments and primary closure of the flap; (**c**) post-op 2 weeks of undisturbed early peri-implant mucosal healing; (**d**) buccal view of the site at second-stage surgery; and (**e**) at post-op 2 weeks

3.1.3 Immune Responses to Biofilm Accumulation Around Implants

The nature of the peri-implant mucosa being exposed to the external and internal environment constitutes a challenge for the immune system to keep the homeostasis between oral microbial stimuli and an appropriate immune response. The lack of the periodontal ligament around implants creates a variety of biological disadvantages for the implant, compared to the periodontium of natural teeth including less physical barrier and reduced blood flow. Periodontal ligament provides the necessary biological niche for the production of immune cells and supports alveolar bone regeneration possibly via the presence of stem-like cells and epithelial cell rests of Malassez [40, 41]. Earlier studies in animal models seem to substantiate this theory that increased bone loss and osteoclasts in ligature-induced peri-implantitis related to the absence of periodontal ligament but not the cervical cementum in cynomolgus monkeys [42].

Biofilm formation in a newly exposed implant can happen as quick as 30 min from the existing species in the oral cavity [43]. Biofilm seems to be confined to the supra-mucosal area with the existence of a plaque and cell-free zone [12]. Similar to gingival tissue, peri-implant mucosa harbor various features that help controlling biofilms including the flushing action of peri-implant crevicular fluid, the rapid epithelial turnover, an influx of innate immune response cells to the peri-implant tissue and the transmigration of neutrophils into the peri-implant sulcus [44, 45]. Stages of inflammatory events are described based on cellular and structural changes occurring during peri-implant mucositis development and progression in experimental studies. A prolonged exposure of the implant site to dental biofilms may induce both qualitative and quantitative changes of the inflammatory infiltrate around peri-implant mucosa, which is reversible upon reinstitution of plaque control similar to those in experimental gingivitis [46]. This response seems to be independent of implant type, at least based on experimental animal models [47]. The sequence of inflammatory events that take place in peri-implant mucositis is similar to those in experimental gingivitis, but potentially of inflammation border extends faster toward the alveolar bone [48]. In humans, experimental peri-implant mucositis lesion at 3 weeks is characterized by the presence of an inflammatory cell infiltrate within the connective tissue underlying oral epithelium [49]. The size of inflammatory lesion around the peri-implant mucosa can reach up to 0.14 mm^2, which is represented by increased proportions of T- and B lymphocytes [50].

The host response patterns in human peri-implantitis are qualitatively similar, yet more extensive, compared to periodontitis, resulting in a faster progression of tissue destruction [51, 52]. The information available on host-immune characteristics of peri-implantitis is derived from comparative studies using biopsy material from peri-implant mucosa and gingiva, as well as experimental studies in animal models. The switch to peri-implantitis from peri-implant mucositis is accompanied by a further influx of inflammatory cells into the affected area of the peri-implant mucosa, that now expands to reach the bone tissue [53, 54] (Fig. 3.5). Similar to advanced periodontitis lesion, apical migration of junctional epithelium, loss of collagen and a larger proportion of neutrophils, macrophages, T- and B-cells, osteoclasts as well as bone loss are the key features of peri-implantitis lesions. When quantified, the size of peri-implantitis lesion is double in size than periodontitis lesion (3.5 vs. 1.5 mm^2) [55]. Diseased tissue obtained from peri-implantitis sites is shown to exhibit higher expression of several mediators of inflammation,

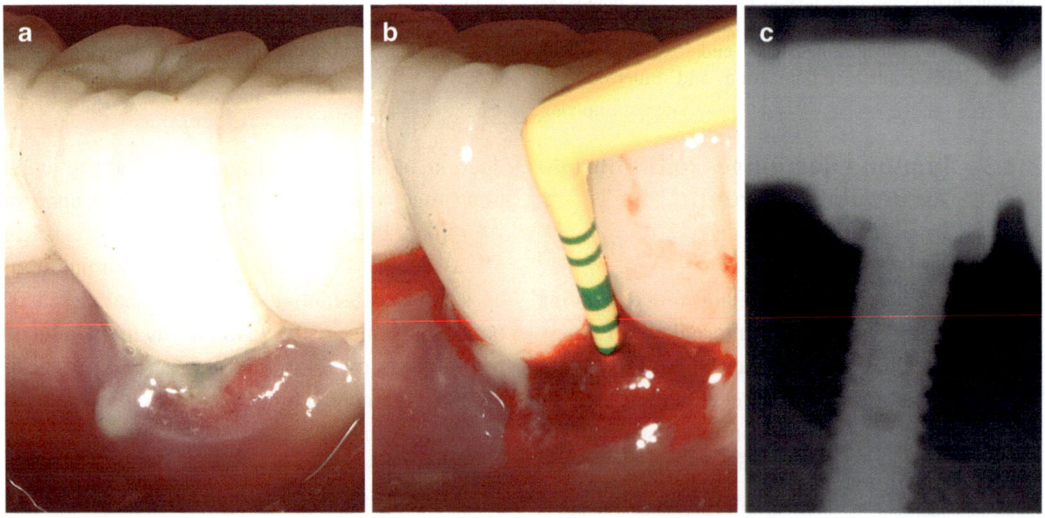

Fig. 3.5 Clinical and radiographic findings of a peri-implantitis case. (**a**) Presence of visual inflammatory changes around the peri-implant soft tissue evident by redness, swelling, ulceration, and suppuration. (**b**) Presence of bleeding on probing, increased probing depth and pus around the implant-supported prosthetic restoration. (**c**) Radiographic evidence of bone loss beyond crestal bone level around the implant

including pro-inflammatory cytokines interleukin (IL)-6, IL-8, and TNF-α, compared to healthy or peri-implant mucositis sites [56, 57]. A global gene expression profiling of peri-implant and gingival mucosa biopsies indicates that both shared and distinct mRNA expression patterns between peri-implantitis and periodontitis. Another high-throughput gene expression study by Liu et al. showed that the cyclooxygenase-2 pathway is the most upregulated biological process in peri-implantitis as compared to periodontitis. Their data also suggested that osteoclast differentiation-related pathways are comparatively more active in peri-implantitis indicated by higher receptor activator of NF-κB (RANK) ligand (RANKL) and osteoprotegerin ratio [58, 59].

Although limited animal models are available to compare peri-implantitis to periodontitis, it's in parallel condition, ligature models in beagle dogs and murine are the most studied ones [60, 61]. The placement of the ligature on the implants of experimental animals results in acute inflammatory reactions that involve tissue breakdown and bone loss, which resemble peri-implantitis in humans [62]. In general, ligatured-induced peri-implantitis presents with increased infiltration of T- and B-cells, neutrophils and macrophages and osteoclasts, while decreased the density of alveolar bone without "self-limiting" process [42, 54, 63–67]. In these models, after the removal of the ligatures, if plaque accumulation is allowed, progression of peri-implantitis occurs resembling natural history of periimplantitis in humans [68]. The lesions in ligatured-induced peri-implantitis appear earlier than they are in periodontitis. By placing ligatures in both tooth and implants of mice for 1 week, 1 month, or 3 months, Hiyari S et al. observed the more intensive bone loss lessons on peri-implantitis compared with periodontitis sites as early as 1 week, and this trend was intensified at later stages [64]. Interestingly, in murine ligature models, at 3 months, 20% of implants exfoliated due to peri-implantitis, but no natural teeth exfoliated in the case of periodontitis [66]. Additionally, removal of ligature leads to bone apposition in periodontitis cases whereas this is not the case in the peri-implantitis group [69]. At the molecular level, increased matrix metalloproteinase-8 (MMP-8), and nuclear factor kappa-light-chain-enhancer of activated B cells (NF-κB) expression seem to follow histopathological observations [64]. Experimental models using knockout mice strains suggested that in toll-like receptor (TLR) 2 and TLR4 mediate bone loss around implants [65, 70]. Similar models were also applied to evaluate the effect of implant type and implant surface characteristics in mediating immune response. The implants with doxycycline-treated surfaces resulted in significantly higher bone levels than the control surface in the peri-implantitis mice model, which showed this surface attenuated inflammatory response and progression [71]. In contrast, implant abutments with antibacterial coating or surface modification with a monolayer of multi-phosphonate molecules in beagle dogs do not seem to prevent biofilm formation on the implant surfaces and do not attenuate host response in the adjacent peri-implant mucosa [72, 73].

3.1.4 Biological Fluids as a Reservoir of Inflammatory Mediators for Peri-Implant Mucositis and Peri-Implantitis and Their Diagnostic Potential

Although histopathologically peri-implant lesions are quite well described, the molecular determinants of these processes are not yet fully described. As indicated by many clinical studies that periodontal indices are not reliable diagnostic and prognostic tools for examining dental implants and determining treatment needs. Although probing clinical pocket depth, clinical attachment level and bleeding on probing (absence or presence) have been recognized as the dentist's most important tools in diagnosing periodontal health and disease, but probing depth around the implants is not as meaningful a diagnostic tool as the tooth. Regular probing around healthy implants could potentially result in trauma to the peri-implant soft tissues with consequent induced inflammation. Therefore, in current practice, probing around dental implants

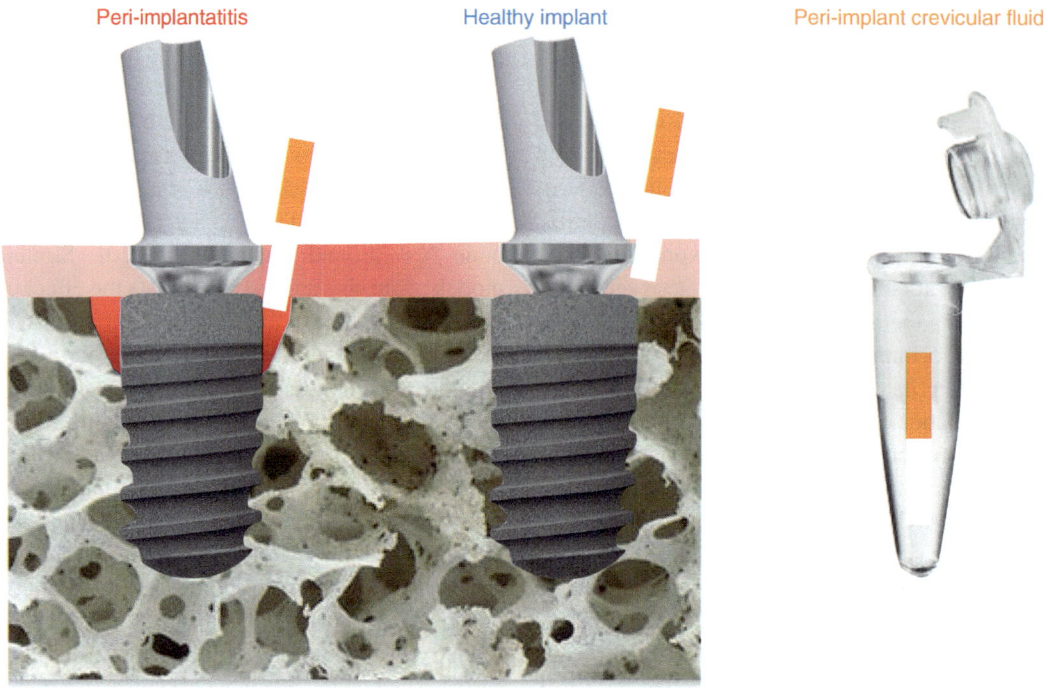

Fig. 3.6 Peri-implant crevicular fluid (PICF) collection in health and disease. The PICF is collected via paper strips after gentle insertion into the crevice for typically 30 s. Once the PICF is absorbed onto the paper strips, then eluted into buffer prior to analysis of the immunological content

cannot be performed until osseointegration is complete which may take up to 6 months [74]. Moreover, probing accuracy is more questionable around peri-implant mucosa as penetration seems to be more advanced at implants than at teeth [63, 75].

Presence bleeding in probing (BOP) around implants is also a poor indicator of progressive peri-implantitis, as BOP is constant both at sites with peri-mucositis and peri-implantitis or even stable peri-implantitis [76]. Ericsson et al. also reported the presence of BOP for the majority of the healthy peri-implant sites [76] potentially indicating a state of subclinical chronic inflammation in healthy peri-implant tissues. Therefore, contemporary, non-invasive diagnostic and prognostic tools based on "measurable biological indicators" of peri-implant diseases are needed to detect active disease and future disease progression and facilitate targeted treatment on a more rational basis. Peri-implant crevicular Fluid (PICF) and saliva are among the proximal sources of biomarkers for peri-implant health and disease. Both saliva and PICF can be obtained non-invasively in less than 5 min (Fig. 3.6). A narrative summary of the literature examining biomarkers in PICF, saliva, and in serum as potential diagnostic/prognostic tools for peri-implant diseases is provided in the following sections.

3.1.5 Peri-Implant Crevicular Fluid

The peri-implant crevicular fluid (PICF) is the inflammatory exudate of the peri-implant sulcus [14, 44]. Similarly, to gingival crevicular fluid (GCF), PICF is the outcome of increased permeability of the vessels within the underlying connective tissue, as an inflammatory response to the growing biofilm at the implant–tissue interface [77]. PICF is enriched with connective tissue breakdown products and inflammatory molecules [78–81]. Therefore, analysis of the PICF might be suitable to evaluate the inflammatory status of peri-implant tissues, in a quantitative manner [45, 82].

In healthy implant tissues, the flow of PICF is minimum. However, in peri-implant mucositis and peri-implantitis, its volume is increased at a given site in response to biofilm accumulation [83, 84]. PICF protein content increases in experimentally induced peri-implant mucositis by the end of the 3 weeks and more interestingly, its volume is higher when compared with that of GCF [48]. Since the composition of PICF is modified along with the histopathological changes during the course of progressive peri-implant inflammation, its molecular analysis may support the early detection of clinically undetectable diseases [85]. The levels of pro-inflammatory cytokines including tumor necrosis factor alpha (TNF-α), Interleukin-1alpha, IL-1 beta (IL-1β) are increased in PICF collected from peri-implantitis-affected sites, compared to healthy controls or sites with periodontitis [86–90]. Further studies also showed that peri-implantitis treatment reduced the PICF levels of IL-1β [91] and TNF-α [92, 93]. Matrix metalloproteinases (MMPs) or their tissue inhibitors (TIMPs) are also found in high levels in PICF from peri-implantitis sites are elevated compared to healthy sites, and their enzymatic activity increases with disease severity or at sites with progressive bone loss risk [89, 94]. The regulation of osteoclastogenesis and osteogenesis-associated markers has also been studied in PICF [95, 96]. Similar to findings in GCF obtained from sites with periodontitis, there is increasing evidence for the association of the RANKL and its inhibitor OPG with the presence and severity of peri-implantitis [48, 97–100]. Higher PICF levels of cathepsin K, a collagenase that is mainly expressed by osteoclasts, have been shown to be associated with peri-implantitis [95, 96, 101]. Although further studies are needed, the current evidence suggests that the assessment of pro-inflammatory cytokines, that is, IL-1β, TNFα, MMP-8, or alveolar bone turnover/resorption molecules, that is, RANKL/OPG or Cathepsin-K in the PICF may be of value as predictors of peri-implant diseases.

3.1.6 Saliva

As an alternative to peri-implant crevicular fluid (PICF), saliva might be used to study host responses against dental implants. Saliva, a complex biofluid composed of minor and major salivary gland secretions, serum and salivary inflammatory mediators and components from the oral microflora, has the potential to reflect oral and systemic health and diseases and can be obtained noninvasively and in large quantities [102, 103]. Various pro- and anti-inflammatory molecules, proteolytic enzymes involved in tissue breakdown as well as markers for bone resorption have been studied in saliva in response to dental implants [104–113].

Significantly higher levels of IL-1β, IL-6, TNF-α, and procalcitonin were present in the saliva of individuals with peri-implantitis compared to healthy controls, and also peri-implant mucositis for procalcitonin [105, 107]. In addition, bleeding on probing positively correlated with salivary procalcitonin in peri-implantitis patients [6, 107]. On the contrary, levels of colony-stimulating factor 1 (CSF-1), IL-34, IL-1β, triggering receptor expressed on myeloid cells (TREM)-1, peptidoglycan recognition protein (PGLYRP)-1, MMP-8, tissue inhibitor of metalloproteinases (TIMP)-1 and MMP-8/TIMP1 ratio in saliva did not differ between peri-implantitis and peri-implant mucositis [9, 12, 110, 113]. Furthermore, CSF-1 in saliva and PICF were positively correlated. Both studies also evaluated the effect of concomitant periodontitis, resulting in significantly higher salivary levels of MMP-8 with both diseases present compared to peri-implantitis alone, while salivary levels of all other molecules were not affected. Furthermore, IL-1β levels in saliva of peri-implant mucositis patients with or without a previous history of periodontitis did not differ [5, 106]. However, in peri-implant mucositis patients without a previous exposure to periodontitis, salivary IL-1β predicted higher levels of IL-1β levels in PICF. Another study investigated peri-implant mucositis patients under regular peri-implant and periodontal therapy or not (controls) at baseline and 5 years after implant placement [108].

Salivary TNF-α was significantly elevated in patients without regular maintenance compared to patients under regular therapy, while IL-1β, IL-10, MMP-2/TIMP-2 complex, Receptor activator of nuclear factor-κB (RANK), osteoprotegerin (OPG), transforming growth factor (TGF)-β did not show any differences.

In a proof-of-concept study, a chewing gum detector was evaluated for its potential to measure MMP-8 activity in saliva by a peptide sensor which when cleaved releases a bitter substance [10, 111]. A significantly higher MMP-8 activity was detected in saliva from peri-implantitis and peri-implant mucositis patients compared to healthy controls. On the contrary, a commercial MMP-8 activity assay used as a control assay was not able to distinguish between healthy and diseased. Furthermore, a pilot study investigated pathogenic gene sets in the saliva of individuals with implant failure due to severe peri-implantitis using a whole-exome sequencing approach [109]. Significant enrichments were identified in gene sets for cytoskeleton, cell adhesion, and metal ion binding. The latter was also identified as a central functional group which, if misregulated, could interfere with cell morphology and adhesion and finally lead to implant failure.

Further studies investigated the host responses to restored and functional implants in the presence and absence of systemic diseases such as obesity [104] or type II diabetes [112]. Salivary IL-1β and IL-6 levels, as well as mean plaque, bleeding on probing, probing depth scores, and bone loss were significantly higher in obese than nonobese men [104]. The study on type II diabetes used an array-based multiplex assay to assess multiple inflammatory molecules at the same time, including IL-1b, IL-2, IL-4, IL-6, IL-8, IL-10, TNF-α, interferon (INF)-γ, C-reactive protein (CRP), macrophage inflammatory protein (MIP)-1α, MIP-1β, MMP-1, MMP-2, MMP-8, MMP-9, TIMP-1, TIMP-2, OPG, adiponectin, and procalcitonin (ProCT) [11, 112]. Salivary markers were measured at baseline and 1 year after implant placement and did not show big differences between the diseased and healthy groups. In patients with type II diabetes, IL-4, IL-10, and OPG were significantly decreased at the 1-year follow-up compared to baseline, while in healthy controls OPG was significantly increased after 1 year compared to baseline. Furthermore, in type II diabetes patients compared to healthy controls, OPG levels were already significantly higher at baseline. None of the other molecules were significantly affected.

3.1.7 Serum

The investigation of health and disease biomarkers in the blood is a standard method, but trends are turning towards other biofluids than blood such as saliva, which can be collected noninvasively and does not require specially trained personnel [103]. However, even though most inflammatory molecules in blood also seem to be detectable in saliva, the concentration of those molecules in the saliva is often substantially lower which might be due to the fluctuating salivary flow rate depending on the circadian rhythm [102, 103]. Hence, investigating the host response to dental implants using whole blood, serum, or plasma should not be neglected. Various studies, as described above for saliva, have investigated inflammatory molecules, proteolytic enzymes, and bone resorption markers in the blood in response to dental biofilm-driven peri-implantitis [112, 114, 115]. A cohort of patients with either successfully osseointegrated dental implants or with dental implants that failed to osseointegrate was investigated for serum IgG to *Actinomyces viscosus*, *Bacteroides forsythus*, *Porphyromonas gingivalis*, *Staphylococcus aureus,* and *Streptococcus intermedius* [13]. Patients with failed implants presented with significantly lower levels of IgG to *S. aureus*, *P. gingivalis,* and *B. forsythus* compared to individuals with successful implants. Furthermore, patients with at least one failed dental implant due to pain, implant movement, or peri-implantitis were tested for IL-1 polymorphisms in the blood [115]. Six out of the 22 patients tested positive for the IL-1 genotype, but the genotype (IL-1 positive or IL-1 negative) did not differentially affect implant failure. However, in smokers, a positive IL-1 genotype resulted in a significantly higher implant failure rate compared to IL-1 positive non-smokers. The study mentioned above investigating the host responses in saliva to functional implants in type II diabetes also analyzed the same molecules in serum at baseline and 1 year after implant placement by using an array-based multiplex assay [112]. Among all molecules, differences were only seen for serum MMP-1, which was significantly higher in healthy controls than type II diabetes patients.

References

1. Williams DF. Specifications for innovative, enabling biomaterials based on the principles of biocompatibility mechanisms. Front Bioeng Biotechnol. 2019;7:255.
2. Williams D. Revisiting the definition of biocompatibility. Med Device Technol. 2003;14(8):10–3.
3. Schroeder A, van der Zypen E, Stich H, Sutter F. The reactions of bone, connective tissue, and epithelium to endosteal implants with titanium-sprayed surfaces. J Maxillofac Surg. 1981;9(1):15–25.
4. Bosshardt DD, Salvi GE, Huynh-Ba G, Ivanovski S, Donos N, Lang NP. The role of bone debris in early healing adjacent to hydrophilic and hydrophobic implant surfaces in man. Clin Oral Implants Res. 2011;22(4):357–64.
5. Berglundh T, Abrahamsson I, Lang NP, Lindhe J. De novo alveolar bone formation adjacent to endosseous implants. Clin Oral Implants Res. 2003;14(3):251–62.
6. Eriksson C, Lausmaa J, Nygren H. Interactions between human whole blood and modified TiO_2-surfaces: influence of surface topography and oxide thickness on leukocyte adhesion and activation. Biomaterials. 2001;22(14):1987–96.
7. Abrahamsson I, Berglundh T, Linder E, Lang NP, Lindhe J. Early bone formation adjacent to rough and turned endosseous implant surfaces. An experimental study in the dog. Clin Oral Implants Res. 2004;15(4):381–92.
8. Trindade R, Albrektsson T, Wennerberg A. Current concepts for the biological basis of dental implants: foreign body equilibrium and osseointegration dynamics. Oral Maxillofac Surg Clin North Am. 2015;27(2):175–83.
9. Maenpaa J, Soderstrom KO, Salmi T, Ekblad U. Large atypical polyps of the vagina during pregnancy with concomitant human papilloma virus infection. Eur J Obstet Gynecol Reprod Biol. 1988;27(1):65–9.
10. Ivanovski S, Hamlet S, Salvi GE, Huynh-Ba G, Bosshardt DD, Lang NP, et al. Transcriptional profiling of osseointegration in humans. Clin Oral Implants Res. 2011;22(4):373–81.
11. Donos N, Hamlet S, Lang NP, Salvi GE, Huynh-Ba G, Bosshardt DD, et al. Gene expression profile of osseointegration of a hydrophilic compared with a hydrophobic microrough implant surface. Clin Oral Implants Res. 2011;22(4):365–72.
12. Tomasi C, Tessarolo F, Caola I, Piccoli F, Wennstrom JL, Nollo G, et al. Early healing of peri-implant mucosa in man. J Clin Periodontol. 2016;43(10):816–24.
13. Gurkan A, Tekdal GP, Bostanci N, Belibasakis GN. Cytokine, chemokine, and growth factor levels in peri-implant sulcus during wound healing and osseointegration after piezosurgical versus conventional implant site preparation: randomized, controlled, split-mouth trial. J Periodontol. 2019;90(6):616–26.
14. Peker Tekdal G, Bostanci N, Belibasakis GN, Gurkan A. The effect of piezoelectric surgery implant osteotomy on radiological and molecular parameters of peri-implant crestal bone loss: a randomized, controlled, split-mouth trial. Clin Oral Implants Res. 2016;27(5):535–44.
15. Ozturk VO, Emingil G, Bostanci N, Belibasakis GN. Impact of implant-abutment connection on osteoimmunological and microbiological parameters in short implants: a randomized controlled clinical trial. Clin Oral Implants Res. 2017;28(9):e111–e20.
16. Hotchkiss KM, Reddy GB, Hyzy SL, Schwartz Z, Boyan BD, Olivares-Navarrete R. Titanium surface characteristics, including topography and wettability, alter macrophage activation. Acta Biomater. 2016;31:425–34.
17. Alfarsi MA, Hamlet SM, Ivanovski S. The effect of platelet proteins released in response to titanium implant surfaces on macrophage pro-inflammatory cytokine gene expression. Clin Implant Dent Relat Res. 2015;17(6):1036–47.
18. Wang Y, Zhang Y, Sculean A, Bosshardt DD, Miron RJ. Macrophage behavior and interplay with gingival fibroblasts cultured on six commercially available titanium, zirconium, and titanium-zirconium dental implants. Clin Oral Investig. 2019;23(8):3219–27.
19. Hotchkiss KM, Ayad NB, Hyzy SL, Boyan BD, Olivares-Navarrete R. Dental implant surface chemistry and energy alter macrophage activation in vitro. Clin Oral Implants Res. 2017;28(4):414–23.
20. Albrektsson T, Dahlin C, Jemt T, Sennerby L, Turri A, Wennerberg A. Is marginal bone loss around oral implants the result of a provoked foreign body reaction? Clin Implant Dent Relat Res. 2014;16(2):155–65.
21. Trindade R, Albrektsson T, Galli S, Prgomet Z, Tengvall P, Wennerberg A. Osseointegration and foreign body reaction: titanium implants activate the immune system and suppress bone resorption during the first 4 weeks after implantation. Clin Implant Dent Relat Res. 2018;20(1):82–91.
22. Young CW, Lee JS, Le H, Smith RA. Surrogate markers of health after titanium dental implant placement. J Oral Maxillofac Surg. 2004;62(11):1413–7.

23. Thomas P, Iglhaut G, Wollenberg A, Cadosch D, Summer B. Allergy or tolerance: reduced inflammatory cytokine response and concomitant IL-10 production of lymphocytes and monocytes in symptom-free titanium dental implant patients. Biomed Res Int. 2013;2013:539834.
24. Quabius ES, Ossenkop L, Harder S, Kern M. Dental implants stimulate expression of Interleukin-8 and its receptor in human blood—an in vitro approach. J Biomed Mater Res B Appl Biomater. 2012;100(5):1283–8.
25. Harder S, Quabius ES, Ossenkop L, Mehl C, Kern M. Surface contamination of dental implants assessed by gene expression analysis in a whole-blood in vitro assay: a preliminary study. J Clin Periodontol. 2012;39(10):987–94.
26. Harder S, Quabius ES, Meinke F, Mehl C, Kern M. Changes in proinflammatory gene expression in human whole blood after contact with UV-conditioned implant surfaces. Clin Oral Investig. 2019;23(10):3731–8.
27. Albrektsson T, Buser D, Sennerby L. Crestal bone loss and oral implants. Clin Implant Dent Relat Res. 2012;14(6):783–91.
28. Kotsakis GA, Olmedo DG. Peri-implantitis is not periodontitis: scientific discoveries shed light on microbiome-biomaterial interactions that may determine disease phenotype. Periodontol 2000. 2021;86(1):231–40.
29. Pettersson M, Kelk P, Belibasakis GN, Bylund D, Molin Thoren M, Johansson A. Titanium ions form particles that activate and execute interleukin-1beta release from lipopolysaccharide-primed macrophages. J Periodontal Res. 2017;52(1):21–32.
30. Olmedo D, Fernandez MM, Guglielmotti MB, Cabrini RL. Macrophages related to dental implant failure. Implant Dent. 2003;12(1):75–80.
31. Tatarakis N, Bashutski J, Wang HL, Oh TJ. Early implant bone loss: preventable or inevitable? Implant Dent. 2012;21(5):379–86.
32. Atieh MA, Alsabeeha NHM, Tawse-Smith A, Duncan WJ. Piezoelectric versus conventional implant site preparation: a systematic review and meta-analysis. Clin Implant Dent Relat Res. 2018;20(2):261–70.
33. Capelli M. Surgical, biologic and implant-related factors affecting bone remodeling around implants. Eur J Esthet Dent. 2013 Summer;8(2):279–313. PMID: 23712347.
34. Berglundh T, Abrahamsson I, Welander M, Lang NP, Lindhe J. Morphogenesis of the peri-implant mucosa: an experimental study in dogs. Clin Oral Implants Res. 2007;18(1):1–8.
35. Tomasi C, Tessarolo F, Caola I, Wennstrom J, Nollo G, Berglundh T. Morphogenesis of peri-implant mucosa revisited: an experimental study in humans. Clin Oral Implants Res. 2014;25(9):997–1003.
36. Araujo MG, Lindhe J. Peri-implant health. J Periodontol. 2018;89(Suppl 1):S249–S56.
37. Berglundh T, Lindhe J, Jonsson K, Ericsson I. The topography of the vascular systems in the periodontal and peri-implant tissues in the dog. J Clin Periodontol. 1994;21(3):189–93.
38. Emecen-Huja P, Eubank TD, Shapiro V, Yildiz V, Tatakis DN, Leblebicioglu B. Peri-implant versus periodontal wound healing. J Clin Periodontol. 2013;40(8):816–24.
39. Khoury SB, Thomas L, Walters JD, Sheridan JF, Leblebicioglu B. Early wound healing following one-stage dental implant placement with and without antibiotic prophylaxis: a pilot study. J Periodontol. 2008;79(10):1904–12.
40. Xiong J, Gronthos S, Bartold PM. Role of the epithelial cell rests of Malassez in the development, maintenance and regeneration of periodontal ligament tissues. Periodontol 2000. 2013;63(1):217–33.
41. Eggert FM, Levin L. Biology of teeth and implants: host factors—pathology, regeneration, and the role of stem cells. Quintessence Int. 2018;49(6):497–509.
42. Schou S, Holmstrup P, Reibel J, Juhl M, Hjorting-Hansen E, Kornman KS. Ligature-induced marginal inflammation around osseointegrated implants and ankylosed teeth: stereologic and histologic observations in cynomolgus monkeys (Macaca fascicularis). J Periodontol. 1993;64(6):529–37.
43. Furst MM, Salvi GE, Lang NP, Persson GR. Bacterial colonization immediately after installation on oral titanium implants. Clin Oral Implants Res. 2007;18(4):501–8.
44. Belibasakis GN, Charalampakis G, Bostanci N, Stadlinger B. Peri-implant infections of oral biofilm etiology. Adv Exp Med Biol. 2015;830:69–84.
45. Belibasakis GN. Microbiological and immuno-pathological aspects of peri-implant diseases. Arch Oral Biol. 2014;59(1):66–72.
46. Liljenberg B, Gualini F, Berglundh T, Tonetti M, Lindhe J. Composition of plaque-associated lesions in the gingiva and the peri-implant mucosa in partially edentulous subjects. J Clin Periodontol. 1997;24(2):119–23.
47. Abrahamsson I, Berglundh T, Lindhe J. Soft tissue response to plaque formation at different implant systems. A comparative study in the dog. Clin Oral Implants Res. 1998;9(2):73–9.
48. Salvi GE, Aglietta M, Eick S, Sculean A, Lang NP, Ramseier CA. Reversibility of experimental peri-implant mucositis compared with experimental gingivitis in humans. Clin Oral Implants Res. 2012;23(2):182–90.
49. Heitz-Mayfield LJA, Salvi GE. Peri-implant mucositis. J Periodontol. 2018;89(Suppl 1):S257–S66.
50. Heitz-Mayfield LJA, Salvi GE. Peri-implant mucositis. J Clin Periodontol. 2018;45(Suppl 20):S237–S45.
51. Dionigi C, Larsson L, Carcuac O, Berglundh T. Cellular expression of DNA damage/repair and reactive oxygen/nitrogen species in human periodontitis and peri-implantitis lesions. J Clin Periodontol. 2020;47(12):1466–75.

52. Charalampakis G, Abrahamsson I, Carcuac O, Dahlen G, Berglundh T. Microbiota in experimental periodontitis and peri-implantitis in dogs. Clin Oral Implants Res. 2014;25(9):1094–8.
53. Gualini F, Berglundh T. Immunohistochemical characteristics of inflammatory lesions at implants. J Clin Periodontol. 2003;30(1):14–8.
54. Lindhe J, Berglundh T, Ericsson I, Liljenberg B, Marinello C. Experimental breakdown of peri-implant and periodontal tissues. A study in the beagle dog. Clin Oral Implants Res. 1992;3(1):9–16.
55. Carcuac O, Berglundh T. Composition of human peri-implantitis and periodontitis lesions. J Dent Res. 2014;93(11):1083–1088.
56. Duarte PM, de Mendonca AC, Maximo MB, Santos VR, Bastos MF, Nociti Junior FH. Differential cytokine expressions affect the severity of peri-implant disease. Clin Oral Implants Res. 2009;20(5):514–20.
57. Venza I, Visalli M, Cucinotta M, De Grazia G, Teti D, Venza M. Proinflammatory gene expression at chronic periodontitis and peri-implantitis sites in patients with or without type 2 diabetes. J Periodontol. 2010;81(1):99–108.
58. Liu Y, Liu Q, Li Z, Acharya A, Chen D, Chen Z, et al. Long non-coding RNA and mRNA expression profiles in peri-implantitis vs periodontitis. J Periodontal Res. 2020;55(3):342–53.
59. Belibasakis GN, Reddi D, Bostanci N. Porphyromonas gingivalis induces RANKL in T-cells. Inflammation. 2011;34(2):133–8.
60. Becker ST, Foge M, Beck-Broichsitter BE, Gavrilova O, Bolte H, Rosenstiel P, et al. Induction of periimplantitis in dental implants. J Craniofac Surg. 2013;24(1):e15–8.
61. Zitzmann NU, Berglundh T, Ericsson I, Lindhe J. Spontaneous progression of experimentally induced periimplantitis. J Clin Periodontol. 2004;31(10):845–9.
62. Schwarz F, Herten M, Sager M, Bieling K, Sculean A, Becker J. Comparison of naturally occurring and ligature-induced peri-implantitis bone defects in humans and dogs. Clin Oral Implants Res. 2007;18(2):161–70.
63. Schou S, Holmstrup P, Stoltze K, Hjorting-Hansen E, Fiehn NE, Skovgaard LT. Probing around implants and teeth with healthy or inflamed peri-implant mucosa/gingiva. A histologic comparison in cynomolgus monkeys (Macaca fascicularis). Clin Oral Implants Res. 2002;13(2):113–26.
64. Hiyari S, Wong RL, Yaghsezian A, Naghibi A, Tetradis S, Camargo PM, et al. Ligature-induced peri-implantitis and periodontitis in mice. J Clin Periodontol. 2018;45(1):89–99.
65. Yu X, Hu Y, Freire M, Yu P, Kawai T, Han X. Role of toll-like receptor 2 in inflammation and alveolar bone loss in experimental peri-implantitis versus periodontitis. J Periodontal Res. 2018;53(1):98–106.
66. Hiyari S, Naghibi A, Wong R, Sadreshkevary R, Yi-Ling L, Tetradis S, et al. Susceptibility of different mouse strains to peri-implantitis. J Periodontal Res. 2018;53(1):107–16.
67. Carcuac O, Abrahamsson I, Albouy JP, Linder E, Larsson L, Berglundh T. Experimental periodontitis and peri-implantitis in dogs. Clin Oral Implants Res. 2013;24(4):363–71.
68. Albouy JP, Abrahamsson I, Persson LG, Berglundh T. Spontaneous progression of ligatured induced peri-implantitis at implants with different surface characteristics. An experimental study in dogs II: histological observations. Clin Oral Implants Res. 2009;20(4):366–71.
69. Wong RL, Hiyari S, Yaghsezian A, Davar M, Casarin M, Lin YL, et al. Early intervention of peri-implantitis and periodontitis using a mouse model. J Periodontol. 2018;89(6):669–79.
70. Deng S, Hu Y, Zhou J, Wang Y, Wang Y, Li S, et al. TLR4 mediates alveolar bone resorption in experimental peri-implantitis through regulation of CD45(+) cell infiltration, RANKL/OPG ratio, and inflammatory cytokine production. J Periodontol. 2020;91(5):671–82.
71. Ding L, Zhang P, Wang X, Kasugai S. A doxycycline-treated hydroxyapatite implant surface attenuates the progression of peri-implantitis: a radiographic and histological study in mice. Clin Implant Dent Relat Res. 2019;21(1):154–9.
72. Almohandes A, Abrahamsson I, Dahlen G, Berglundh T. Effect of biofilm formation on implant abutments with an anti-bacterial coating: a pre-clinical in vivo study. Clin Oral Implants Res. 2021;32(6):756–66.
73. Sanz-Esporrin J, Di Raimondo R, Pla R, Luengo F, Vignoletti F, Nunez J, et al. Experimental peri-implantitis around titanium implants with a chemically modified surface with a mono-layer of multi-phosphonate molecules: a pre-clinical in vivo investigation. Clin Oral Investig. 2021;25(6):3789–800.
74. Serino G, Turri A, Lang NP. Probing at implants with peri-implantitis and its relation to clinical peri-implant bone loss. Clin Oral Implants Res. 2013;24(1):91–5.
75. Lang NP, Wetzel AC, Stich H, Caffesse RG. Histologic probe penetration in healthy and inflamed peri-implant tissues. Clin Oral Implants Res. 1994;5(4):191–201.
76. Lekholm U, Adell R, Lindhe J, Branemark PI, Eriksson B, Rockler B, et al. Marginal tissue reactions at osseointegrated titanium fixtures. (II) A cross-sectional retrospective study. Int J Oral Maxillofac Surg. 1986;15(1):53–61.
77. Bostanci N, Belibasakis GN. Gingival crevicular fluid and its immune mediators in the proteomic era. Periodontol 2000. 2018;76(1):68–84.
78. Adonogianaki E, Mooney J, Wennstrom JL, Lekholm U, Kinane DF. Acute-phase proteins and immunoglobulin G against Porphyromonas gingivalis in peri-implant crevicular fluid: a comparison

with gingival crevicular fluid. Clin Oral Implants Res. 1995;6(1):14–23.
79. Kaklamanos EG, Tsalikis L. A review on peri-implant crevicular fluid assays potential in monitoring and predicting peri-implant tissue responses. J Int Acad Periodontol. 2002;4(2):49–59.
80. Golub LM, Raisanen IT, Sorsa T, Preshaw PM. An unexplored pharmacologic/diagnostic strategy for peri-implantitis: a protocol proposal. Diagnostics (Basel). 2020;10(12)
81. Thierbach R, Maier K, Sorsa T, Mantyla P. Peri-implant sulcus fluid (PISF) matrix metalloproteinase (MMP) -8 levels in peri-implantitis. J Clin Diagn Res. 2016;10(5):ZC34–8.
82. Esberg A, Isehed C, Holmlund A, Lundberg P. Peri-implant crevicular fluid proteome before and after adjunctive enamel matrix derivative treatment of peri-implantitis. J Clin Periodontol. 2019;46(6):669–77.
83. Guncu GN, Akman AC, Gunday S, Yamalik N, Berker E. Effect of inflammation on cytokine levels and bone remodelling markers in peri-implant sulcus fluid: a preliminary report. Cytokine. 2012;59(2):313–6.
84. Schierano G, Pejrone G, Brusco P, Trombetta A, Martinasso G, Preti G, et al. TNF-alpha TGF-beta2 and IL-1beta levels in gingival and peri-implant crevicular fluid before and after de novo plaque accumulation. J Clin Periodontol. 2008;35(6):532–8.
85. Schincaglia GP, Hong BY, Rosania A, Barasz J, Thompson A, Sobue T, et al. Clinical, immune, and microbiome traits of gingivitis and peri-implant mucositis. J Dent Res. 2017;96(1):47–55.
86. Curtis DA, Kao R, Plesh O, Finzen F, Franz L. Crevicular fluid analysis around two failing dental implants: a clinical report. J Prosthodont. 1997;6(3):210–4.
87. Severino VO, Napimoga MH, de Lima Pereira SA. Expression of IL-6, IL-10, IL-17 and IL-8 in the peri-implant crevicular fluid of patients with peri-implantitis. Arch Oral Biol. 2011;56(8):823–8.
88. Alassy H, Parachuru P, Wolff L. Peri-implantitis diagnosis and prognosis using biomarkers in peri-implant crevicular fluid: a narrative review. Diagnostics (Basel). 2019;9(4)
89. Wang HL, Garaicoa-Pazmino C, Collins A, Ong HS, Chudri R, Giannobile WV. Protein biomarkers and microbial profiles in peri-implantitis. Clin Oral Implants Res. 2016;27(9):1129–36.
90. Recker EN, Avila-Ortiz G, Fischer CL, Pagan-Rivera K, Brogden KA, Dawson DV, et al. A cross-sectional assessment of biomarker levels around implants versus natural teeth in periodontal maintenance patients. J Periodontol. 2015;86(2):264–72.
91. Bassetti M, Schar D, Wicki B, Eick S, Ramseier CA, Arweiler NB, et al. Anti-infective therapy of peri-implantitis with adjunctive local drug delivery or photodynamic therapy: 12-month outcomes of a randomized controlled clinical trial. Clin Oral Implants Res. 2014;25(3):279–87.
92. de Mendonca AC, Santos VR, Cesar-Neto JB, Duarte PM. Tumor necrosis factor-alpha levels after surgical anti-infective mechanical therapy for peri-implantitis: a 12-month follow-up. J Periodontol. 2009;80(4):693–9.
93. Faot F, Nascimento GG, Bielemann AM, Campao TD, Leite FR, Quirynen M. Can peri-implant crevicular fluid assist in the diagnosis of peri-implantitis? A systematic review and meta-analysis. J Periodontol. 2015;86(5):631–45.
94. Arakawa H, Uehara J, Hara ES, Sonoyama W, Kimura A, Kanyama M, et al. Matrix metalloproteinase-8 is the major potential collagenase in active peri-implantitis. J Prosthodont Res. 2012;56(4):249–55.
95. Strbac GD, Monov G, Cei S, Kandler B, Watzek G, Gruber R. Cathepsin K levels in the crevicular fluid of dental implants: a pilot study. J Clin Periodontol. 2006;33(4):302–8.
96. Yamalik N, Gunday S, Kilinc K, Karabulut E, Berker E, Tozum TF. Analysis of cathepsin-K levels in biologic fluids from healthy or diseased natural teeth and dental implants. Int J Oral Maxillofac Implants. 2011;26(5):991–7.
97. Rakic M, Lekovic V, Nikolic-Jakoba N, Vojvodic D, Petkovic-Curcin A, Sanz M. Bone loss biomarkers associated with peri-implantitis. A cross-sectional study. Clin Oral Implants Res. 2013;24(10):1110–6.
98. Bostanci N, Saygan B, Emingil G, Atilla G, Belibasakis GN. Effect of periodontal treatment on receptor activator of NF-kappaB ligand and osteoprotegerin levels and relative ratio in gingival crevicular fluid. J Clin Periodontol. 2011;38(5):428–33.
99. Reddi D, Bostanci N, Hashim A, Aduse-Opoku J, Curtis MA, Hughes FJ, et al. Porphyromonas gingivalis regulates the RANKL-OPG system in bone marrow stromal cells. Microbes Infect. 2008;10(14–15):1459–68.
100. Rakic M, Struillou X, Petkovic-Curcin A, Matic S, Canullo L, Sanz M, et al. Estimation of bone loss biomarkers as a diagnostic tool for peri-implantitis. J Periodontol. 2014;85(11):1566–74.
101. Yamalik N, Gunday S, Uysal S, Kilinc K, Karabulut E, Tozum TF. Analysis of cathepsin-K activity at tooth and dental implant sites and the potential of this enzyme in reflecting alveolar bone loss. J Periodontol. 2012;83(4):498–505.
102. Lee YH, Wong DT. Saliva: an emerging biofluid for early detection of diseases. Am J Dent. 2009;22(4):241–8.
103. Castagnola M, Scarano E, Passali GC, Messana I, Cabras T, Iavarone F, et al. Salivary biomarkers and proteomics: future diagnostic and clinical utilities. Acta Otorhinolaryngol Ital. 2017;37(2):94–101.
104. Abduljabbar T, Al-Sahaly F, Kellesarian SV, Kellesarian TV, Al-Anazi M, Al-Khathami M, et al. Comparison of peri-implant clinical and radiographic inflammatory parameters and whole salivary destructive inflammatory cytokine pro-

file among obese and non-obese men. Cytokine. 2016;88:51–6.
105. Abduljabbar T, Vohra F, Ullah A, Alhamoudi N, Khan J, Javed F. Relationship between self-rated pain and peri-implant clinical, radiographic and whole salivary inflammatory markers among patients with and without peri-implantitis. Clin Implant Dent Relat Res. 2019;21(6):1218–24.
106. Acharya A, Koh ML, Kheur S, Watt RM, Jin L, Mattheos N. Salivary IL-1beta and red complex bacteria as predictors of the inflammatory status in sub-peri-implant niches of subjects with peri-implant mucositis. Clin Oral Implants Res. 2016;27(6):662–7.
107. Algohar A, Alqerban A. Levels of procalcitonin in saliva and peri-implant crevicular fluid in patients with peri-implant diseases and health. Arch Oral Biol. 2020;120:104931.
108. Gomes AM, Douglas-de-Oliveira DW, Ferreira SD, Silva TAD, Cota LOM, Costa FO. Periodontal disease, peri-implant disease and levels of salivary biomarkers IL-1beta, IL-10, RANK, OPG, MMP-2, TGF-beta and TNF-alpha: follow-up over 5 years. J Appl Oral Sci. 2019;27:e20180316.
109. Lee S, Kim JY, Hwang J, Kim S, Lee JH, Han DH. Investigation of pathogenic genes in peri-implantitis from implant clustering failure patients: a whole-exome sequencing pilot study. PLoS One. 2014;9(6):e99360.
110. Lira-Junior R, Teixeira MKS, Lourenco EJV, Telles DM, Figueredo CM, Bostrom EA. CSF-1 and IL-34 levels in peri-implant crevicular fluid and saliva from patients having peri-implant diseases. Clin Oral Investig. 2020;24(1):309–15.
111. Ritzer J, Luhmann T, Rode C, Pein-Hackelbusch M, Immohr I, Schedler U, et al. Diagnosing peri-implant disease using the tongue as a 24/7 detector. Nat Commun. 2017;8(1):264.
112. Tatarakis N, Kinney JS, Inglehart M, Braun TM, Shelburne C, Lang NP, et al. Clinical, microbiological, and salivary biomarker profiles of dental implant patients with type 2 diabetes. Clin Oral Implants Res. 2014;25(7):803–12.
113. Teixeira MKS, Lira-Junior R, Lourenco EJV, Telles DM, Bostrom EA, Figueredo CM, et al. The modulation of the TREM-1/PGLYRP1/MMP-8 axis in peri-implant diseases. Clin Oral Investig. 2020;24(5):1837–44.
114. Kronstrom M, Svensson B, Erickson E, Houston L, Braham P, Persson GR. Humoral immunity host factors in subjects with failing or successful titanium dental implants. J Clin Periodontol. 2000;27(12):875–82.
115. Jansson H, Hamberg K, De Bruyn H, Bratthall G. Clinical consequences of IL-1 genotype on early implant failures in patients under periodontal maintenance. Clin Implant Dent Relat Res. 2005;7(1):51–9.

In Vitro and In Vivo Models to Understand Biofilm Implant Infections

4

Syatirah-Najmi Abdullah and Nicholas S. Jakubovics

4.1 Introduction

Improvements in oral health rely on the development and implementation of new ideas and approaches including behavioural interventions, drugs or medical devices such as dental implants. The translational pathway from idea to implementation is long and complex. For new drugs and medical devices, it is essential to demonstrate safety and efficacy in preclinical models before moving to clinical trials. Models can also be used to screen compound libraries and identify promising drug candidates as well as to define the mechanism of action underpinning new therapies. Highly simplified models have advantages such as ease of use, low cost, high throughput and high measurement accuracy. However, simple models do not replicate the highly complex biology of the human body. Therefore, multiple models will be needed to fully characterise a new agent. It is essential to select the most appropriate model for the research question. This chapter describes some of the key models that have been used to investigate biofilm infections on and around dental implants.

4.1.1 Key Characteristics of Peri-Implant Biofilms

A good model will replicate the biological system as closely as possible while allowing opportunities to assess the impact of interventions on different aspects of the system and providing sufficient simplification to enable detailed measurements of system parameters. Before developing a model, it is essential to consider the key characteristics of the system to be modelled. Biofilm formation on and around dental implants has been described earlier in this book. The system is highly complex in terms of both the microbiology and the surrounding environment of host tissues. The microbiome varies according to health/disease status (Table 4.1) and in all cases, there is a complex microbial biofilm present with multiple species of bacteria [1]. The biofilm is embedded in a matrix of polymers that includes extracellular DNA and polysaccharides [2, 3]. During implant healing and in peri-implant disease, the biofilm is bathed in gingival crevicular fluid and contains host inflammatory cells and cytokines [4, 5]. Environmental factors such as smoking affect the composition of the peri-implant biofilm [6, 7]. When developing a model, it is essential to consider which aspects of the

S.-N. Abdullah
Faculty of Dentistry, Universiti Sains Islam Malaysia, Kuala Lumpur, Malaysia
e-mail: najmi@usim.edu.my

N. S. Jakubovics (✉)
School of Dental Sciences, Faculty of Medical Sciences, Newcastle University, Newcastle upon Tyne, UK
e-mail: nick.jakubovics@newcastle.ac.uk

P. Neelakantan, A. Princy Solomon (eds.), *Dental Implants and Oral Microbiome Dysbiosis*,
https://doi.org/10.1007/978-3-030-99014-5_4

Table 4.1 Key bacterial taxa enriched in peri-implant health or disease[a]

Health	Peri-mucositis	Peri-implantitis
Neisseria spp.	*Porphyromonas* spp.	*Porphyromonas gingivalis*
Streptococcus sanguinis	*Tannerella forsythia*	*Porphyromonas endodontalis*
Streptococcus intermedius	*Treponema denticola*	*Tannerella forsythia*
Corynebacterium matruchotii	*Prevotella* spp.	*Fusobacterium nucleatum*
Rothia spp.	*Fusobacterium* spp.	*Fretibacterium fastidiosum*
Capnocytophaga spp.	*Streptococcus* spp.	*Prevotella intermedia*
Veillonella spp.	*Leptotrichia* spp.	*Treponema* spp.
Lautropia mirabilis	*Peptostreptococcaceae* XIG-5	*Filifactor alocis*
Granulicatella spp.	*Selenomonas* spp.	*Desulfobulbus* sp.
Actinomyces spp.	*Ottowia* sp.	
Lactobacillus spp.	*Lachnospiraceae* [G-3]	
	Clostridiales [F-2][G-1]	

[a]Data were extracted from the following references: [4, 8–14]

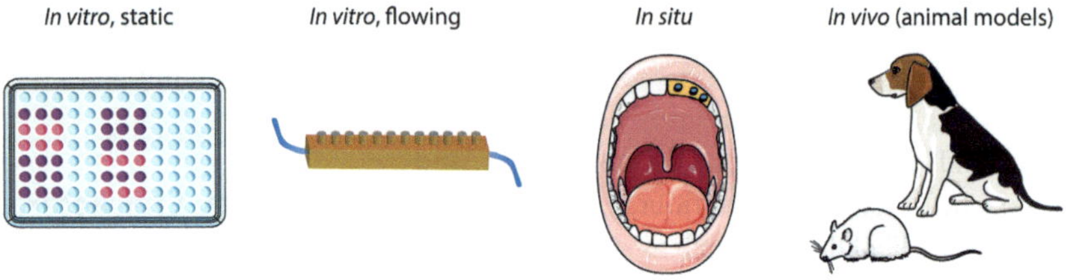

Cost	Low	Low/medium	Medium	High
Throughput	High	Medium	Low	Low
Complexity/relevance	Low	Low/medium	High	High
Interventions	Possible	Possible	Difficult*	Possible
Ethical issues	None#	None#	Discomfort/health	Animal welfare
Uses	Screening	Advanced screening	Natural biofilm analysis	Advanced testing

Fig. 4.1 Overview of models for biofilm analysis. Models need to be selected according to the intended use. Initial screening of biofilm growth or antibiofilm compounds may use high-throughput in vitro static models such as the microtitre plate system. More robust biofilms can be grown in flowing systems such as the Modified Robbins device. Biofilms grown in situ, for example, on a piece of enamel held within an intraoral stent, will most closely mimic natural dental plaque. Animal models may be required to assess toxicity or efficacy of materials including implants. *Interventions such as the application of drugs are usually not possible within in situ models, but may be applied after the biofilm is removed from the mouth. #Ethical issues for in vitro models may arise if the model incorporates body fluids such as saliva or serum. This figure includes artwork from Servier Medical Art (https://smart.servier.com/)

microbiome, host cells and tissues and environmental factors need to be incorporated.

The host tissue environment surrounding implants can only be replicated with in vivo animal models. However, there is a drive to reduce the use of animal models for ethical reasons and because findings in animals often do not replicate those in humans [15]. Appropriate in vitro models have advantages over in vivo models including reduced cost and increased reproducibility (Fig. 4.1). In situ models such as enamel chips held within stents in the mouths of volunteers can be used to replicate the growth of biofilms in the mouth. Although it is not possible to challenge these biofilms in situ with products that have not yet received regulatory approval, some models allow removal of the biofilms and assessment of responses in vitro. In general, simple in vitro models with high throughput and low cost are excellent for early-stage research such as the screening of compound libraries or biofilm formation capacity of microbes. Further characterisation requires more complex in vitro models. Due to the complexity of the implant environment, animal models are still required for a more detailed understanding of the interactions between biofilm and host.

4.1.2 In Vitro Model Systems

4.1.2.1 Static Models

The simplest model systems involve a defined inoculum such as a single species of bacteria, an inert surface and a rich medium to ensure the strong growth of the biofilm. Microtitre plates with 96 wells provide a simple, economical system for evaluating biofilm growth. Following incubation of microorganisms in the growth medium, biofilms are formed on the surface of the wells or in a ring around the air-liquid interface and can be stained with crystal violet to quantify the level of biomass formed [16]. However, it is well-recognised that stochastic variation from handling and processing samples can affect the conclusions drawn from the crystal violet biofilm assay and is therefore recommended that this is not used for detailed characterisation of biofilm formation [17]. One concern with the microtitre plate system is that biofilm formation may be affected by the settling of microbes due to gravity. To ameliorate this issue, models have been developed to grow biofilms on vertical surfaces such as pegs attached to the lid of the plate (the Calgary biofilm device) or discs of different materials suspended in clamps fitted to a custom-made lid of a 24-well plate (the active attachment biofilm model) [18, 19].

Criteria for defining medically relevant biofilms include both structural characteristics and increased recalcitrance to antimicrobial agents [20]. Staining with crystal violet provides little information about either of these. Instead, indicators of metabolic activity can be employed to understand the vitality of the biofilm. For example, tetrazolium salts such as 3-(4,5-dimethylthia zol-2-yl)-2,5-diphenyl tetrazolium bromide (MTT) or 2,3-Bis-(2-Methoxy-4-Nitro-5-Sulfop henyl)-2H-Tetrazolium-5-Carboxanilide (XTT) provide a colour change when they are reduced by metabolically active cells [21, 22]. In addition, live:dead staining can highlight specific locations where bacteria in a biofilm are inactivated by antimicrobial treatments [23]. The direct visualisation of biofilm in microwell plates requires either a relatively large well with a dipping lens or an optically clear glass bottom placed on an inverted microscope [24]. Alternatively, biofilms may be cultured on removable inserts within the microplate to facilitate microscopy. Confocal laser scanning microscopy (CLSM) has become the method of choice for biofilm visualisation since it can provide three-dimensional structural information in combination with fluorescent dyes and without any requirement for dehydrating the samples (Fig. 4.2a). Structural parameters of biofilms can then be quantified with software packages such as COMSTAT2, daime, BiofilmQ or BAIT [25–28]. However, for high-resolution images of biofilms, tools such as scanning electron microscopy (SEM) are required. In our experience, field emission SEM provides excellent structural detail of bacterial cells and matrix material (Fig. 4.2b), although it is important to note that the matrix is inevitably collapsed due to dehydration during sample processing [29]. Three-dimensional SEM approaches involving sequential imaging of slices produced by a microtome embedded in the microscope (Fig. 4.2c) or ablation of the surface by a focused ion beam can provide high-resolution structural information on microbial communities [30, 31].

4.1.2.2 Models with Fluid Flow

The major nutrient sources for oral biofilms, saliva or GCF, continuously flow into and out of the mouth. This creates additional sheer forces over the biofilms and, perhaps more importantly, leads to a continual replenishment of nutrients and removal of waste products. The incorporation of flow is a key feature of many in vitro biofilm model systems. There are three main approaches to deliver fluid flow: (i) drip feed into the system and over the biofilm samples, (ii) culture biofilms in stirred vessels, with nutrients added and removed at a constant rate and (iii) direct flow over the biofilms. Examples of each approach are shown in Fig. 4.3.

Drip feed systems are designed to culture biofilms under a thin film of liquid, replicating the conditions found on the exposed surfaces of teeth. This can be achieved simply by dripping growth medium onto the upper end of a microscope slide that has been tilted at an angle. A chamber for simultaneously culturing multiple

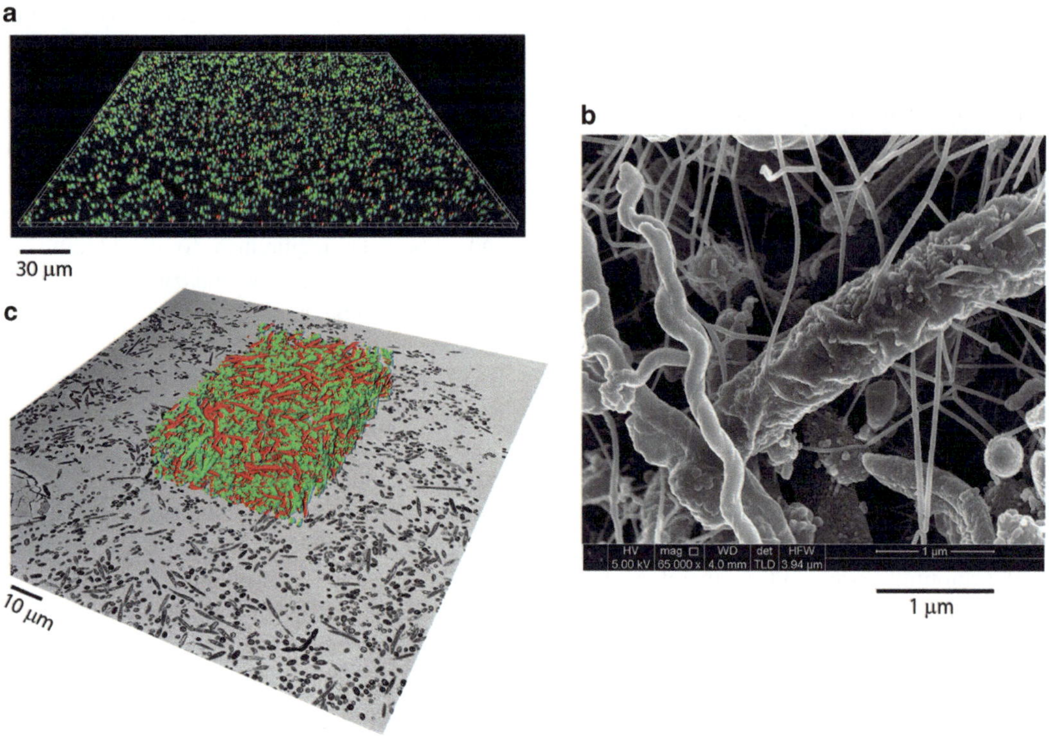

Fig. 4.2 Microscopy approaches for biofilm visualisation. (**a**) *Staphylococcus aureus* biofilm visualised by CLSM with live:dead staining. Viable cells are stained with Syto9 and appear green. Compromised cells stained with propidium iodide appear red. (**b**) Field emission SEM image of subgingival dental plaque, showing thin strings of biofilm matrix material. (**c**) Three-dimensional SEM reconstruction of a dual-species biofilm containing *Streptococcus gordonii* (artificially coloured green based on cell shape) and *Fusobacterium nucleatum* (coloured red)

biofilms has been developed and is a recognised standard test method for the quantification of *Pseudomonas aeruginosa* biofilms [32–34]. This approach has been used in oral microbiology, for example, to assess chlorhexidine tolerance in dual-species biofilms containing *Streptococcus mutans* and *Actinomyces naeslundii* [35]. The Constant Depth Film Fermenter (CDFF) also supplies nutrients by dripping them into the reactor vessel, but in this system, the biofilm samples are held horizontally (Fig. 4.3a) [36, 37]. The CDFF was originally developed by Julian Wimpenny and colleagues in the 1980s in order to culture biofilms in a steady-state and at a constant depth to provide a robust system for monitoring responses of a well-defined biofilm to perturbations [38]. Biofilm samples are held in pans that are recessed to a fixed depth (300 µm in the original design). Liquid drips into the system over paddles that scrape across the biofilm samples, which are continuously rotated by a motor underneath the system. Although long-term steady-state biofilms are difficult to achieve, the fluid flow characteristics and the ability to culture multiple biofilms within a single vessel make this system well-suited to longitudinal studies of oral biofilm formation. One disadvantage is that all samples within a CDFF vessel have the same exposure so parallel experiments require multiple vessels, which are costly and technically challenging to set up. Nevertheless, it has been shown that CDFF vessels run in parallel have good levels of reproducibility for culturing oral microcosm biofilms [39].

An alternative to culturing biofilms in steady state is to grow them on coupons immersed in a more traditional fermenter, in which the free-living (planktonic) cells are in steady-state growth. For example, a two-stage chemostat system has been described for the culture of a 10-membered oral

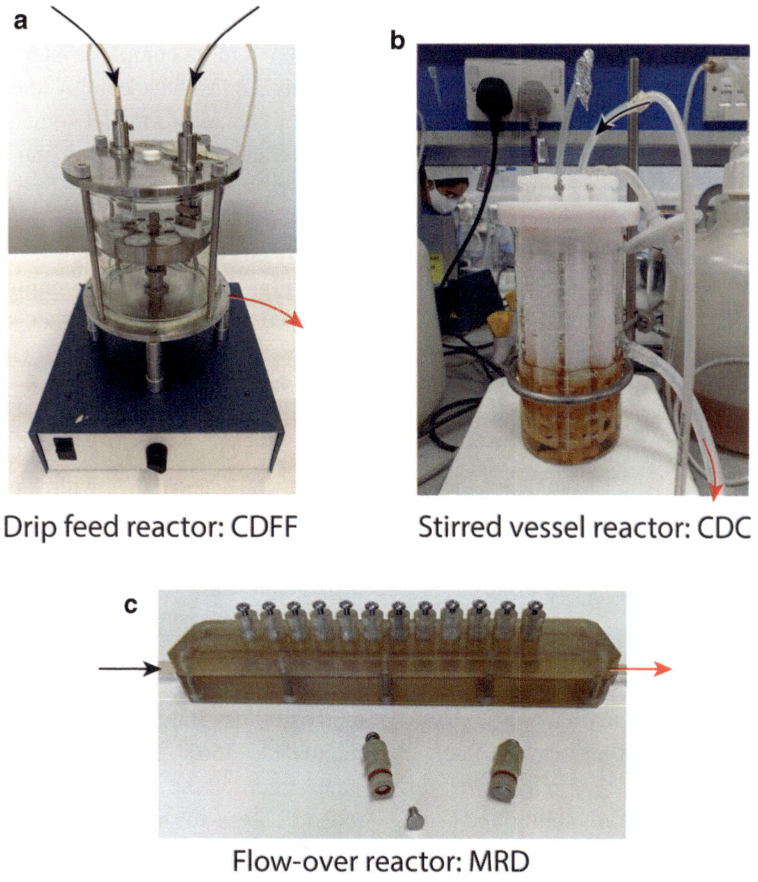

Fig. 4.3 Examples of biofilm reactors that incorporate flow. (**a**) The constant depth film fermenter (CDFF) drips medium onto paddles that scrape over the surface of the biofilm holders. Biofilms are grown on surfaces recessed at a fixed depth. The lower part of the system incorporates a motor that rotates the biofilm sample holders, ensuring they are continuously scraped by the paddle. (**b**) The CDC biofilm reactors are stirred vessels that contain biofilm samples in specialised holders. (**c**) The Modified Robbins Device (MRD) contains samples set flush against the walls of a tube. Medium is directly flowed over the samples. The direction of flow into the vessels is shown as black arrows and flow out of the systems is indicated by red arrows. In each case, fluid flow is driven by pumps (not shown)

biofilm community [40]. In this model, the first chemostat was used to obtain steady-state planktonic growth before the second-stage chemostat, containing suspended biofilm coupons, was attached to the outflow. A simpler single-stage chemostat specifically designed to hold biofilm coupons, known as the CDC Biofilm Reactor®, is commercially available from BioSurface Technologies, Bozeman, MT, USA (Fig. 4.3b). This is a relatively controllable system that is well-suited to assessing biofilm growth on dental materials or in dental unit waterlines [41, 42].

Many biofilm models simply flow growth medium directly over the substratum to culture biofilms within the channel of the device. For example, the Modified Robbins Device (MRD) is designed to hold removable sample discs of different materials flush against the wall of the vessel (Fig. 4.3c) [43]. This system provides a relatively large channel and can be used for culturing mixed-species oral biofilms that produce extensive polysaccharides which would block smaller systems [44]. Parallel MRD chambers enable comparisons of biofilm formation under different conditions and the presence of multiple sampling ports allows repeated biofilm sampling and analysis during longitudinal studies. However, it is important to note that a gradient of adhesion may be present along the device and sampling strategies should take this into account

[45]. In addition, the MRD does not permit real-time visualisation of biofilm growth or removal. This requires systems such as the flow-cell that culture biofilms on transparent cover glass [46]. Like the MRD, flow cells contain a central channel through which the growth medium is pumped. Comparisons between different treatments require multiple channels or flow cells run in parallel. The relatively small dimensions of the flow-cell make it realistic to use diluted human saliva as a growth medium for biofilms, replicating the conditions present in the mouth [46]. However, to run flow cells overnight usually requires more than 100 mL of human saliva. To reduce the need for saliva collection from volunteers, miniaturised systems such as the BioFlux microfluidics model have been employed to culture oral biofilms [47].

4.1.2.3 Importance of the Inoculum

Oral biofilms typically contain tens or hundreds of different species of bacteria, with viruses, Archaea and single-celled eukaryotes such as fungi and/or protozoa. Models often aim for simplification to increase reproducibility and facilitate analytical approaches. Some bacteria will form monospecies biofilms in vitro that allow the dissection of molecular pathways involved in surface attachment and colonisation. *P. aeruginosa* has become the model of choice for many biofilm studies due to its clinical relevance in cystic fibrosis, burn and wound infections, its genetic tractability and its ability to form structured biofilms [48]. However, *P. aeruginosa* is not a major constituent of dental plaque, except perhaps in certain populations [49, 50]. *Streptococcus mutans* is more commonly used as a target for assessing biofilm control agents due to its strong association with dental caries [51]. Biofilm formation by *S. mutans* is highly dependent on the presence of sucrose, which is utilised by extracellular glucosyltransferase and fructosyltransferase enzymes for the production of exopolysaccharides [52]. By contrast, *Enterococcus faecalis*, a persistent coloniser in root canal infections, produces biofilm matrix enriched in extracellular DNA [53]. Although extracellular matrix is readily observed in *E. faecalis* monospecies biofilms, it is difficult to replicate the dense cell–cell interactions observed in more complex systems (Fig. 4.4).

Many studies have employed defined communities of bacteria to model some of the interspecies interactions that occur in oral biofilms. When members of the community form clearly distinct cell shapes, it may be possible to distinguish them by SEM or other high-resolution microscopy (Fig. 4.4b). Selective culture can also be employed where the appropriate selective agents are known [54]. A quantitative PCR approach has been used to enumerate different species in a 14-member community [55]. This study employed a DNA cross-linking dye to bind extracellular DNA and DNA within non-viable cells so that only viable bacteria were quantified. In theory, similar approaches can be combined with deep sequencing to quantify the viable microbiome of any microbial system. However, caution is warranted with this method since complex microbial communities do not respond consistently to cross-linking agents such as propidium monoazide [56]. Nevertheless, more conventional microbiome analysis provides a powerful tool to assess the relative numbers of different taxa and enables a detailed analysis of biofilms containing the natural microbes present in the oral cavity. Consequently, there has been significant interest recently in finding systems that will allow the stable culturing of microcosm biofilm communities isolated from oral health or disease. For example, recent work has shown that saliva supplemented with 5% human serum provides an excellent growth medium for culturing the subgingival microbiota [57].

4.1.2.4 Incorporation of Host Cells and Environmental Factors

The biofilm models described above are designed to model the growth of bacteria on hard surfaces such as human enamel. However, peri-implant biofilms are also in contact with soft tissues. Although it is difficult to achieve stable long-term co-culture of bacteria with soft tissues, models have been developed to challenge cells and tissues with biofilms and biofilm products. For example, studies of invasive infections such as candidiasis have employed organotypic mod-

Fig. 4.4 Levels of microbial complexity in biofilm models visualised by FE-SEM. (**a**) Monospecies biofilms of *E. faecalis* contain extracellular material that appears as strings between the microbial cells. However, cells do not adopt the densely packed arrangements of more complex biofilms. (**b**) A 7 species biofilm including two fungi (*Candida*) and five bacteria isolated from tracheoesophageal speech valves. The bacteria are *Lactobacillus fermentum*, *Streptococcus oralis*, *Ochrobactrum anthropi*, *Staphylococcus aureus* and *Staphylococcus epidermidis*. Different species can be distinguished by their cell shape and arrangement such as *S. oralis* (*So*, strings of cocci), *L. fermentum* (*Lf*, relatively thin rods) or *Candida* (*Ca*/*Cg*, large yeast, pseudohyphae or hyphae). Matrix material is also visible. (**c**) Subgingival dental plaque on a recently-extracted tooth contains many different cells that cannot easily be identified without staining. Extracellular matrix material is abundant

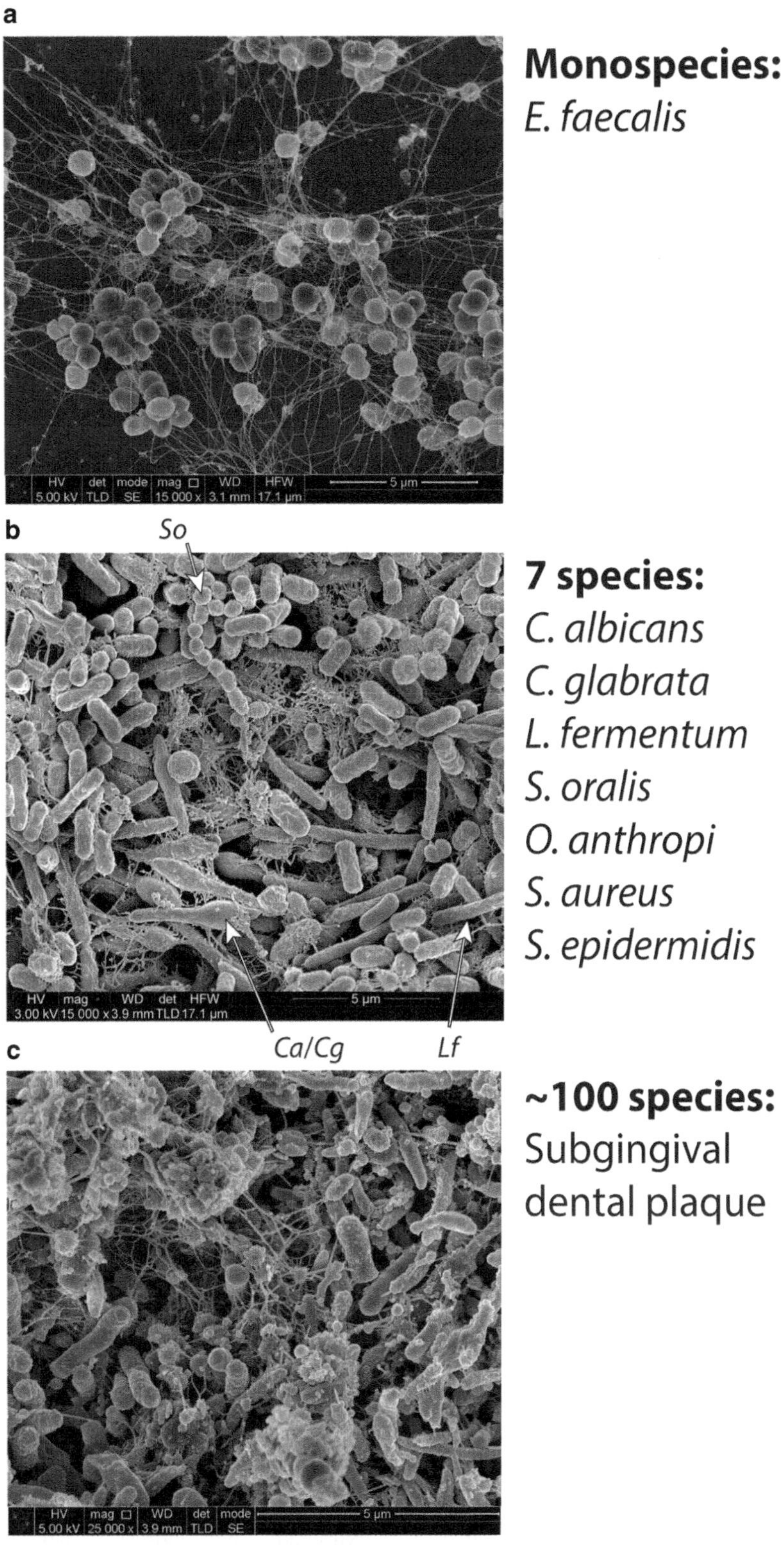

els as substrates for the development of biofilms [58]. Similarly, *Aggregatibacter actinomycetemcomitans* has been shown to reduce the expression of keratin by gingival epithelial cells in an organotypic model of gingival tissue [59]. An alternative approach to investigate biofilm-host interactions is to culture biofilms in a transwell system and apply them to tissue culture cells on the surface of plastic dishes [60]. The use of these and other systems to investigate the immune response to oral biofilms and these have been reviewed in detail recently by Brown et al. [61].

The incorporation of dietary factors into biofilm models is easily achieved by adjusting the growth medium as needed. However, exposure to cigarette smoke and e-cigarette vapour is an important factor for periodontal disease and peri-implantitis that is more difficult to reproduce in the laboratory. The simplest approach is to add tobacco smoke extract, nicotine or e-cigarette liquids to the biofilm growth medium. For example, the addition of cigarette smoke extract to planktonic *Streptococcus gordonii* or *Porphyromonas gingivalis* causes changes in gene expression [62]. More recently, systems have been developed to expose biofilms to smoke or vapour [63]. Exposure to e-cigarette vapour increases the expression of genes encoding glucosyltransferase, competence and glucan-binding proteins and enhances biofilm formation by *S. mutans* [64]. In a more complex model involving mixed-species biofilms and host cells, exposure to tobacco smoke led to enhanced immunogenicity of commensal biofilms, but a dampening down of the inflammatory capacity of pathogen-rich biofilms [65]. Overall, these data highlight the complex interplay between microbes, host and environmental factors that can only be replicated by sophisticated model systems.

4.1.3 In Situ Models

The development of a model to culture marine 'bacterial films' in situ was perhaps the first example of biofilm research [66]. In situ models are also widely used for developing biofilms within the oral cavity that can then be extracted and analysed. A wide range of models have been developed and these have been reviewed elsewhere [67]. Of course, these models are restricted to areas of the mouth that can be accessed without causing harm. Therefore, the majority of in situ models have been developed for studying early microbial colonisation of teeth or the development of cariogenic biofilms. One innovative approach is the development of a combined system that develops biofilms in situ and then utilises a 3D-printed microfluidic flow-cell device to continue culturing biofilms in vitro [68]. This system has been employed to demonstrate the effects of exposing in situ-grown biofilms to sucrose on the pH in different areas of the biofilm. The model could also be employed to challenge natural biofilms with experimental agents that are not yet approved for use in clinical studies.

4.1.4 In Vivo Models

A major limitation of in vitro and in situ models for research on peri-implant biofilms is that they do not include the interaction with alveolar bone that is a critical factor for stabilising the implant. Brånemark introduced the term 'osseointegration', which was initially described as 'a direct structural and functional connection between ordered, living bone and the surface of a load-carrying implant' [69] and later redefined as 'clinical osseointegration implies histologic osseointegration, it is necessary [there is] a contiguous contact between the alveolar bone and the implant surface' [70]. Many factors influence osseointegration such as the implant surface topography, chemical composition and surface roughness [71]. The process of osseointegration is still actively studied as it is not yet fully understood [72].

The use of animal models is the only way currently to include osseointegration in addition to biofilm formation and to translate the experimental knowledge for clinical uses related to dental implant applications. Several different parameters need to be considered such as the variety of dental implants [73] and materials used [74], in addition to the factors that cause implant failure including biofilm formation and treatment [75]. Models may address peri-implant mucositis (inflammatory lesion of the soft tissues around the implant) or peri-implantitis (affecting supporting bone) since both are caused by microbial biofilms. It is important to note that peri-implantitis varies from periodontitis in terms of the rate of progression, the extent of lesion formation and the composition of cells in the lesion [76]. It is still not clear how closely the microbiome of peri-implantitis resembles that of periodontitis, but a review by Rakic et al. [77] suggested that there are common species found in cases of periodontal disease and peri-implant infection, but their microbiome status is not identical.

Previously, many studies modelling peri-implant infections employed large animal models such as dogs and pigs [73, 78, 79]. However, due to housing, ease of handling and commercial availability with different genetic backgrounds, small laboratory animals such as rodents are gaining some interest for implant-associated animal model research [80, 81]. These animal models are induced to form peri-implant infections by various methods such as implantation of a device colonised with a human pathogen [82], split-mouth model [83] or ligatures tied around implants to facilitate the accumulation of bacteria [81].

Ligature-induced defect animal models are employed to mimic a natural peri-implantitis lesion [81, 82, 84]. This technique involves the induction of mucositis and peri-implantitis lesions by the introduction of ligatures around the implant neck in a submucosal position in areas of plaque formation [84]. This experimentally induced invasive procedure is associated with spontaneous disease progression in a majority of sites [79] and is more often employed to study osseointegration than biofilm infection per se [82]. The use of ligatures will initiate an inflammatory response and induce bone destructive processes [85]. Changes in the microbial composition of peri-implant pockets will also be influenced by ligatures [86].

4.1.4.1 Canine Models

Canine models are commonly used to investigate biofilm accumulation and spontaneous periodontitis [87] in studies of dental implant application and its association with peri-implantitis [78]. Human and canine bones possess similarities including bone weight, density and composition and dogs are able to use human-sized implants. However, there are some limitations since the rate of remodelling and apposition may vary within and/ or between dogs [72, 80].

Studies have employed the split-mouth design in a beagle dog model to evaluate peri-implant tissue clinically, radiographically, microbiologically and histologically [83, 88, 89]. In the split-mouth model, each dog hemi-mandible will be randomly assigned by matched pair design to either test implant group or control implant group. To examine the role of oral hygiene, the control implant can be brushed daily while the test implants are left untouched [88]. From this work, the test group had differences in total bacteria, *Fusobacterium* spp., *A. actinomycetemcomitans* and *Porphyromonas gingivalis* and there were significant increases in probing depth, bleeding-on-probing and clinical attachment level versus baseline that were consistent with the onset of peri-implantitis. Furthermore, the split-mouth model adapted from previous studies [83] can also be used for the detection, classification and measurement of peri-implant bone defects. Various analysis methods are available and a recent study has shown advantages of cone beam computed tomography (CBCT) compared with intra-oral (IO) radiography for the assessment of bone defects [89].

4.1.4.2 Rodent Models

Rodent models of polymicrobial peri-implantitis have been used to investigate the inflammatory response to human microbial biofilms [90, 91]. For example, a split-mouth implant model in specific pathogen-free female ex-breeder Sprague-Dawley rats was used to investigate and quantify the implant-associated biofilm. Besides the establishment of a three-step implantation method for titanium implants [92], this model can be excellent for analysing microbial growth when the biofilm formation process is left to occur naturally after the inoculation of human-derived oral bacteria *Streptococcus oralis*, *Fusobacterium nucleatum* and *P. gingivalis* orally [90]. This approach is similar to a previous report that used Wistar rats and established reproducible biofilm quantification using fluorescence staining and confocal scanning laser microscopy [91]. In addition, PCR was used for the identification of microbial taxa present in the samples. A blinded clinical inspection of the implantation site was done by a dentist and any signs of infection were evaluated at the end of the experiment using an established mucosa index based on the gingival index described by Löe [93]. Koutouzis et al. [91] and Sun et al. [75] reported that bacterial colonisation/infection around implants caused significant IgG and IgM antibody responses. There was advanced bone resorption, and extensive inflammation with granulation tissue and PMNs observed in the peri-implantitis model.

The rat model was reported to have 79.6% successful osseous initial integration [90], similar to a report by Koutouzis et al. [91]. This high success rate may be due to the implant assembling steps practised in both studies. This technique overcame problems with the establishment of a direct bone-implant interface reported in previous studies that were caused by movements of the implant during osseous integration [92]. Furthermore, there were signs of mild to moderate peri-implant mucositis in animals with confirmed polymicrobial infection, which were absent in control animals treated with antibiotics [90].

This animal model allows an easy insertion and removal of the implant abutment when needed. This advantage is that this not only protects the abutment from wear and abrasion or unwanted colonisation by endogenous bacteria but also provides the possibility to observe and quantify three-dimensional biofilm formation of this model using confocal scanning laser microscopy of the abutment and retaining screw. Besides the established clinical situation where there is bacterial leakage from the implant-abutment connection, they highlighted that this model still needs a further modification due to the presence of a cavity under the retaining screw that may act as a good hiding place for the biofilm community to form [94, 95].

4.2 Summary

There is still much to learn about the development of microbial biofilms on dental implants and the surrounding tissues. Good model systems are essential for enhancing our understanding of these processes and how to control them. In addition to the in vitro, in situ and in vivo models described here, it is likely that we will see a rapid expansion in the use of in silico models, in part driven by the development of artificial intelligence and deep learning [96]. Ultimately, these models will lead to the development of improved dental implants that provide strength, longevity and that are able to remain free of pathogenic infections over their lifetime of use.

References

1. Belibasakis GN, Manoil D. Microbial community-driven etiopathogenesis of peri-implantitis. J Dent Res. 2021;100(1):21–8.
2. Costa RC, Souza JGS, Bertolini M, Retamal-Valdes B, Feres M, Barão VAR. Extracellular biofilm matrix leads to microbial dysbiosis and reduces biofilm susceptibility to antimicrobials on titanium biomaterial: an in vitro and in situ study. Clin Oral Implants Res. 2020;31(12):1173–86.
3. Rostami N, Shields RC, Yassin SA, Hawkins AR, Bowen L, Luo TL, Rickard AH, Holliday R, Preshaw PM, Jakubovics NS. A critical role for extracellular DNA in dental plaque formation. J Dent Res. 2017;96(2):208–16.
4. Schincaglia GP, Hong BY, Rosania A, Barasz J, Thompson A, Sobue T, Panagakos F, Burleson JA, Dongari-Bagtzoglou A, Diaz PI. Clinical, immune, and microbiome traits of gingivitis and peri-implant mucositis. J Dent Res. 2017;96(1):47–55.
5. Payne JB, Johnson PG, Kok CR, Gomes-Neto JC, Ramer-Tait AE, Schmid MJ, Hutkins RW. Subgingival microbiome colonization and cytokine production during early dental implant healing. mSphere. 2017;2(6)
6. Pimentel SP, Fontes M, Ribeiro FV, Corrêa MG, Nishii D, Cirano FR, MZ C, RCV C. Smoking habit modulates peri-implant microbiome: a case-control study. J Periodontal Res. 2018;53(6):983–91.
7. Tsigarida AA, Dabdoub SM, Nagaraja HN, Kumar PS. The influence of smoking on the peri-implant microbiome. J Dent Res. 2015;94(9):1202–17.
8. Dabdoub SM, Tsigarida AA, Kumar PS. Patient-specific analysis of periodontal and peri-implant microbiomes. J Dent Res. 2013;92(12 Suppl):168s–75s.
9. Ghensi P, Manghi P, Zolfo M, Armanini F, Pasolli E, Bolzan M, Bertelle A, Dell'Acqua F, Dellasega E, Waldner R, et al. Strong oral plaque microbiome signatures for dental implant diseases identified by strain-resolution metagenomics. NPJ Biofilms Microbiomes. 2020;6(1):47.
10. Lu H, Yan X, Zhu B, Zhang L, Feng X, Piao M, Huang B, Wang X, Zhang H, Wang Q, et al. The occurrence of peri-implant mucositis associated with the shift of submucosal microbiome in patients with a history of periodontitis during the first two years. J Clin Periodontol. 2021;48(3):441–54.
11. Martellacci L, Quaranta G, Fancello G, D'Addona A, Sanguinetti M, Patini R, Masucci L. Characterizing

peri-implant and sub-gingival microbiota through culturomics. First isolation of some species in the oral cavity. A pilot study. Pathogens. 2020;9(5)
12. Polymeri A, van der Horst J, Buijs MJ, Zaura E, Wismeijer D, Crielaard W, Loos BG, Laine ML, Brandt BW. Submucosal microbiome of peri-implant sites: a cross-sectional study. J Clin Periodontol. 2021;
13. Sanz-Martin I, Doolittle-Hall J, Teles RP, Patel M, Belibasakis GN, Hämmerle CHF, Jung RE, FRF T. Exploring the microbiome of healthy and diseased peri-implant sites using illumina sequencing. J Clin Periodontol. 2017;44(12):1274–84.
14. Wang Q, Lu H, Zhang L, Yan X, Zhu B, Meng H. Peri-implant mucositis sites with suppuration have higher microbial risk than sites without suppuration. J Periodontol. 2020;91(10):1284–94.
15. Kerecman Myers D, Goldberg AM, Poth A, Wolf MF, Carraway J, McKim J, Coleman KP, Hutchinson R, Brown R, Krug HF, et al. From *in vivo* to *in vitro*: the medical device testing paradigm shift. ALTEX. 2017;34(4):479–500.
16. Merritt JH, Kadouri DE, O'Toole GA. Growing and analyzing static biofilms. Curr Protoc Microbiol. 2005; Chapter 1:Unit 1B.1
17. Kragh KN, Alhede M, Kvich L, Bjarnsholt T. Into the well—a close look at the complex structures of a microtiter biofilm and the crystal violet assay. Biofilms. 2019;1:100006.
18. Ceri H, Olson ME, Stremick C, Read RR, Morck D, Buret A. The calgary biofilm device: new technology for rapid determination of antibiotic susceptibilities of bacterial biofilms. J Clin Microbiol. 1999;37(6):1771–6.
19. Fernandez Y, Mostajo M, Exterkate RAM, Buijs MJ, Beertsen W, van der Weijden GA, Zaura E, Crielaard W. A reproducible microcosm biofilm model of subgingival microbial communities. J Periodontal Res. 2017;52(6):1021–31.
20. Parsek MR, Singh PK. Bacterial biofilms: an emerging link to disease pathogenesis. Annu Rev Microbiol. 2003;57:677–701.
21. Li YY, Li BS, Liu WW, Cai Q, Wang HY, Liu YQ, Liu YJ, Meng WY. Effects of d-arginine on *porphyromonas gingivalis* biofilm. J Oral Sci. 2020;62(1):57–61.
22. Peeters E, Nelis HJ, Coenye T. Comparison of multiple methods for quantification of microbial biofilms grown in microtiter plates. J Microbiol Methods. 2008;72(2):157–65.
23. Takenaka S, Trivedi HM, Corbin A, Pitts B, Stewart PS. Direct visualization of spatial and temporal patterns of antimicrobial action within model oral biofilms. Appl Environ Microbiol. 2008;74(6):1869–75.
24. Rao D, Arvanitidou E, Du-Thumm L, Rickard AH. Efficacy of an alcohol-free cpc containing mouthwash against oral multispecies biofilms. J Clin Dent. 2011;22(6):187–94.
25. Daims H, Lücker S, Wagner M. Daime, a novel image analysis program for microbial ecology and biofilm research. Environ Microbiol. 2006;8(2):200–13.
26. Hartmann R, Jeckel H, Jelli E, Singh PK, Vaidya S, Bayer M, DKH R, Vidakovic L, Díaz-Pascual F, JCN F, et al. Quantitative image analysis of microbial communities with biofilmq. Nat Microbiol. 2021;6(2):151–6.
27. Heydorn A, Nielsen AT, Hentzer M, Sternberg C, Givskov M, Ersboll BK, Molin S. Quantification of biofilm structures by the novel computer program comstat. Microbiology (Reading). 2000;146(Pt 10):2395–407.
28. Luo TL, Hayashi M, Zsiska M, Circello B, Eisenberg M, Gonzalez-Cabezas C, Foxman B, Marrs CF, Rickard AH. Introducing bait (biofilm architecture inference tool): a software program to evaluate the architecture of oral multi-species biofilms. Microbiology (Reading). 2019;165(5):527–37.
29. Holliday R, Preshaw PM, Bowen L, Jakubovics NS. The ultrastructure of subgingival dental plaque, revealed by high-resolution field emission scanning electron microscopy. BDJ Open. 2015;1:15003.
30. Cao Y, Su B, Chinnaraj S, Jana S, Bowen L, Charlton S, Duan P, Jakubovics NS, Chen J. Nanostructured titanium surfaces exhibit recalcitrance towards staphylococcus epidermidis biofilm formation. Sci Rep. 2018;8(1):1071.
31. Mutha NVR, Mohammed WK, Krasnogor N, Tan GYA, Choo SW, Jakubovics NS. Transcriptional responses of *streptococcus gordonii* and *fusobacterium nucleatum* to coaggregation. Mol Oral Microbiol. 2018;33(6):450–64.
32. ASTM Standards. Standard test method for quantification of *pseudomonas aeruginosa* biofilm grown using drip flow biofilm reactor with low shear and continuous flow. West Conshohocken, PA: ASTM International; 2020.
33. Goeres DM, Hamilton MA, Beck NA, Buckingham-Meyer K, Hilyard JD, Loetterle LR, Lorenz LA, Walker DK, Stewart PS. A method for growing a biofilm under low shear at the air-liquid interface using the drip flow biofilm reactor. Nat Protoc. 2009;4(5):783–8.
34. Goeres DM, Parker AE, Walker DK, Meier K, Lorenz LA, Buckingham-Meyer K. Drip flow reactor method exhibits excellent reproducibility based on a 10-laboratory collaborative study. J Microbiol Methods. 2020;174:105963.
35. de Oliveira RVD, Bonafe FSS, Spolidorio DMP, Koga-Ito CY, Farias AL, Kirker KR, James GA, Brighenti FL. *Streptococcus mutans* and *actinomyces naeslundii* interaction in dual-species biofilm. Microorganisms. 2020;8(2)
36. Kinniment SL, Wimpenny JW, Adams D, Marsh PD. The effect of chlorhexidine on defined, mixed culture oral biofilms grown in a novel model system. J Appl Bacteriol. 1996a;81(2):120–5.
37. Kinniment SL, Wimpenny JWT, Adams D, Marsh PD. Development of a steady-state oral microbial biofilm community using the constant-depth film fermenter. Microbiology (Reading). 1996b;142(Pt 3):631–8.

38. Peters AC, Wimpenny JW. A constant-depth laboratory model film fermentor. Biotechnol Bioeng. 1988;32(3):263–70.
39. Hope CK, Bakht K, Burnside G, Martin GC, Burnett G, de Josselin de Jong E, Higham SM. Reducing the variability between constant-depth film fermenter experiments when modelling oral biofilm. J Appl Microbiol. 2012;113(3):601–8.
40. Bradshaw DJ, Marsh PD, Allison C, Schilling KM. Effect of oxygen, inoculum composition and flow rate on development of mixed-culture oral biofilms. Microbiol-UK. 1996;142:623–9.
41. Rudney JD, Chen R, Lenton P, Li J, Li Y, Jones RS, Reilly C, Fok AS, Aparicio C. A reproducible oral microcosm biofilm model for testing dental materials. J Appl Microbiol. 2012;113(6):1540–53.
42. Yoon HY, Lee SY. Establishing a laboratory model of dental unit waterlines bacterial biofilms using a cdc biofilm reactor. Biofouling. 2017;33(10):917–26.
43. Kharazmi A, Giwercman B, Høiby N. [16] robbins device in biofilm research. Methods Enzymol. 1999:207–15.
44. Yassin SA, German MJ, Rolland SL, Rickard AH, Jakubovics NS. Inhibition of multispecies biofilms by a fluoride-releasing dental prosthesis copolymer. J Dent. 2016;48:62–70.
45. Kerr CJ, Jones CR, Hillier VF, Robson GD, Osborn KS, Handley PS. Statistical evaluation of a newly modified robbins device using a bioluminescent pseudomonad to quantify adhesion to plastic. Biofouling. 2000;14(4):267–77.
46. Palmer RJ Jr, Kazmerzak K, Hansen MC, Kolenbrander PE. Mutualism versus independence: strategies of mixed-species oral biofilms in vitro using saliva as the sole nutrient source. Infect Immun. 2001;69(9):5794–804.
47. Samarian DS, Jakubovics NS, Luo TL, Rickard AH. Use of a high-throughput in vitro microfluidic system to develop oral multi-species biofilms. Jove-J Vis Exp. 2014;94
48. Musken M, Di Fiore S, Dotsch A, Fischer R, Haussler S. Genetic determinants of pseudomonas aeruginosa biofilm establishment. Microbiology. 2010;156(Pt 2):431–41.
49. Colombo APV, Tanner ACR. The role of bacterial biofilms in dental caries and periodontal and peri-implant diseases: a historical perspective. J Dent Res. 2019;98(4):373–85.
50. Vieira Colombo AP, Magalhães CB, Hartenbach FA, Martins do Souto R, Maciel da Silva-Boghossian C. Periodontal-disease-associated biofilm: a reservoir for pathogens of medical importance. Microb Pathog. 2016;94:27–34.
51. Lemos JA, Quivey RG, Koo H, Abranches J. *Streptococcus mutans*: a new gram-positive paradigm? Microbiology (Reading). 2013;159(Pt 3):436–45.
52. Koo H, Xiao J, Klein MI, Jeon JG. Exopolysaccharides produced by *streptococcus mutans* glucosyltransferases modulate the establishment of microcolonies within multispecies biofilms. J Bacteriol. 2010;192(12):3024–32.
53. Barnes AM, Ballering KS, Leibman RS, Wells CL, Dunny GM. *Enterococcus faecalis* produces abundant extracellular structures containing DNA in the absence of cell lysis during early biofilm formation. MBio. 2012;3(4):e00193–12.
54. Bradshaw DJ, Marsh PD. Analysis of ph-driven disruption of oral microbial communities in vitro. Caries Res. 1998;32(6):456–62.
55. Chatzigiannidou I, Teughels W, Van de Wiele T, Boon N. Oral biofilms exposure to chlorhexidine results in altered microbial composition and metabolic profile. npj Biofilms Microbiomes. 2020;6(1):13.
56. Wang Y, Yan Y, Thompson KN, Bae S, Accorsi EK, Zhang Y, Shen J, Vlamakis H, Hartmann EM, Huttenhower C. Whole microbial community viability is not quantitatively reflected by propidium monoazide sequencing approach. Microbiome. 2021;9(1):17.
57. Baraniya D, Naginyte M, Chen T, Albandar JM, Chialastri SM, Devine DA, Marsh PD, Al-hebshi NN. Modeling normal and dysbiotic subgingival microbiomes: effect of nutrients. J Dent Res. 2020;99(6):695–702.
58. Sobue T, Bertolini M, Thompson A, Peterson DE, Diaz PI, Dongari-Bagtzoglou A. Chemotherapy-induced oral mucositis and associated infections in a novel organotypic model. Mol Oral Microbiol. 2018;33(3):212–23.
59. Beklen A, Torittu A, Ihalin R, Pöllänen M. *Aggregatibacter actinomycetemcomitans* biofilm reduces gingival epithelial cell keratin expression in an organotypic gingival tissue culture model. Pathogens. 2019;8(4)
60. Millhouse E, Jose A, Sherry L, Lappin DF, Patel N, Middleton AM, Pratten J, Culshaw S, Ramage G. Development of an *in vitro* periodontal biofilm model for assessing antimicrobial and host modulatory effects of bioactive molecules. BMC Oral Health. 2014;14(1):80.
61. Brown JL, Johnston W, Delaney C, Short B, Butcher MC, Young T, Butcher J, Riggio M, Culshaw S, Ramage G. Polymicrobial oral biofilm models: simplifying the complex. J Med Microbiol. 2019;68(11):1573–84.
62. Bagaitkar J, Daep CA, Patel CK, Renaud DE, Demuth DR, Scott DA. Tobacco smoke augments *porphyromonas gingivalis-streptococcus gordonii* biofilm formation. PLoS One. 2011;6(11):e27386.
63. Holliday R, Chaffee BW, Jakubovics NS, Kist R, Preshaw PM. Electronic cigarettes and oral health. J Dent Res. 2021;100(9):906–13.
64. Rouabhia M, Semlali A. Electronic cigarette vapor increases *streptococcus mutans* growth, adhesion, biofilm formation, and expression of the biofilm-associated genes. Oral Dis. 2021;27(3):639–47.
65. Shah SA, Ganesan SM, Varadharaj S, Dabdoub SM, Walters JD, Kumar PS. The making of a miscreant: tobacco smoke and the creation of pathogen-rich biofilms. NPJ Biofilms Microbiomes. 2017;3:26.
66. Zobell CE, Allen EC. The significance of marine bacteria in the fouling of submerged surfaces. J Bacteriol. 1935;29(3):239–51.

67. Prada-Lopez I, Quintas V, Vilaboa C, Suarez-Quintanilla D, Tomas I. Devices for in situ development of non-disturbed oral biofilm. A systematic review. Front Microbiol. 2016;7:1055.
68. Kristensen MF, Leonhardt D, Neland MLB, Schlafer S. A 3d printed microfluidic flow-cell for microscopy analysis of in situ-grown biofilms. J Microbiol Methods. 2020;171:105876.
69. Brånemark PI, Hansson BO, Adell R, Breine U, Lindström J, Hallén O, Ohman A. Osseointegrated implants in the treatment of the edentulous jaw. Experience from a 10-year period. Scand J Plast Reconstr Surg Suppl. 1977;16:1–132.
70. Brånemark PI, Adell R, Albrektsson T, Lekholm U, Lundkvist S, Rockler B. Osseointegrated titanium fixtures in the treatment of edentulousness. Biomaterials. 1983;4(1):25–8.
71. Matos GRM. Surface roughness of dental implant and osseointegration. J Maxillofac Oral Surg. 2021;20(1):1–4.
72. Elias CN, Meirelles L. Improving osseointegration of dental implants. Expert Rev Med Devices. 2010;7(2):241–56.
73. Wancket LM. Animal models for evaluation of bone implants and devices: comparative bone structure and common model uses. Vet Pathol. 2015;52(5):842–50.
74. Brunello G, Biasetto L, Elsayed H, Sbettega E, Gardin C, Scanu A, Carmignato S, Zavan B, Sivolella S. An in vivo study in rat femurs of bioactive silicate coatings on titanium dental implants. J Clin Med. 2020;9(5)
75. Sun J, Eberhard J, Glage S, Held N, Voigt H, Schwabe K, Winkel A, Stiesch M. Development of a peri-implantitis model in the rat. Clin Oral Implants Res. 2020;31(3):203–14.
76. Kantarci A, Hasturk H, Van Dyke TE. Animal models for periodontal regeneration and peri-implant responses. Periodontol. 2015;68(1):66–82.
77. Rakic M, Grusovin MG, Canullo L. The microbiologic profile associated with peri-Implantitis in humans: a systematic review. Int J Oral Maxillofac Implants. 2016;31(2):359–68.
78. Pearce AI, Richards RG, Milz S, Schneider E, Pearce SG. Animal models for implant biomaterial research in bone: a review. Eur Cell Mater. 2007;13:1–10.
79. Schwarz F, Herten M, Sager M, Bieling K, Sculean A, Becker J. Comparison of naturally occurring and ligature-induced peri-implantitis bone defects in humans and dogs. Clin Oral Implants Res. 2007;18(2):161–70.
80. Graves DT, Fine D, Teng Y-TA, Van Dyke TE, Hajishengallis G. The use of rodent models to investigate host–bacteria interactions related to periodontal diseases. J Clin Periodontol. 2008;35(2):89–105.
81. Oz HS, Puleo DA. Animal models for periodontal disease. J Biomed Biotechnol. 2011;2011:754857.
82. Pirih FQ, Hiyari S, Barroso ADV, Jorge ACA, Perussolo J, Atti E, Tetradis S, Camargo PM. Ligature-induced peri-implantitis in mice. J Periodontal Res. 2015;50(4):519–24.
83. Huang Y, Li Z, Van Dessel J, Salmon B, Huang B, Lambrichts I, Politis C, Jacobs R. Effect of platelet-rich plasma on peri-implant trabecular bone volume and architecture: a preclinical micro-ct study in beagle dogs. Clin Oral Implants Res. 2019;30(12):1190–9.
84. Berglundh T, Lindhe J, Marinello C, Ericsson I, Liljenberg B. Soft tissue reaction to de novo plaque formation on implants and teeth. An experimental study in the dog. Clin Oral Implants Res. 1992;3(1):1–8.
85. Pesce P, Menini M, Tealdo T, Bevilacqua M, Pera F, Pera P. Peri-implantitis: a systematic review of recently published papers. Int J Prosthodont. 2014;27(1):15–25.
86. Charalampakis G, Abrahamsson I, Carcuac O, Dahlén G, Berglundh T. Microbiota in experimental periodontitis and peri-implantitis in dogs. Clin Oral Implants Res. 2014;25(9):1094–8.
87. Dard M. 13 - methods and interpretation of performance studies for dental implants. In: Boutrand J-P, editor. Biocompatibility and performance of medical devices. Woodhead Publishing; 2012. p. 308–44.
88. Martins O, Ramos JC, Mota M, Dard M, Viegas C, Caramelo F, Nogueira C, Gonçalves T, Baptista IP. Evaluation of a novel dog animal model for peri-implant disease: clinical, radiographic, microbiological and histological assessment. Clin Oral Investig. 2020;24(9):3121–32.
89. Song D, Shujaat S, de Faria Vasconcelos K, Huang Y, Politis C, Lambrichts I, Jacobs R. Diagnostic accuracy of cbct versus intraoral imaging for assessment of peri-implant bone defects. BMC Med Imaging. 2021;21(1):23.
90. Blank E, Grischke J, Winkel A, Eberhard J, Kommerein N, Doll K, Yang I, Stiesch M. Evaluation of biofilm colonization on multi-part dental implants in a rat model. BMC Oral Health. 2021;21(1):313.
91. Koutouzis T, Eastman C, Chukkapalli S, Larjava H, Kesavalu L. A novel rat model of polymicrobial peri-implantitis: a preliminary study. J Periodontol. 2017;88(2):e32–41.
92. Albrektsson T, Brånemark PI, Hansson HA, Lindström J. Osseointegrated titanium implants: requirements for ensuring a long-lasting, direct bone-to-implant anchorage in man. Acta Orthop Scand. 1981;52(2):155–70.
93. Löe HJTJP. The gingival index, the plaque index and the retention index systems. J Periodontol. 1967;38(6):610–6.
94. Lauritano D, Moreo G, Lucchese A, Viganoni C, Limongelli L, Carinci F. The impact of implant-abutment connection on clinical outcomes and microbial colonization: a narrative review. Materials (Basel, Switzerland). 2020;13(5)
95. Quirynen M, Van Steenberghe D. Bacterial colonization of the internal part of two-stage implants. An in vivo study. Clin Oral Implants Res. 1993;4(3):158–61.
96. Joda T, Yeung AWK, Hung K, Zitzmann NU, Bornstein MM. Disruptive innovation in dentistry: what it is and what could be next. J Dent Res. 2021;100(5):448–53.

Modern Approaches to Biofilm Management on Dental Implants

5

Vinay Sivaswamy and Prasanna Neelakantan

5.1 Modern Approaches to Biofilm Management on Dental Implants

Oral permucosal implants are the current gold standard treatment option for replacing missing teeth. The literature accumulated over the last two decades emphasise the ubiquitous adoption of this treatment option across a multitude of clinical situations, as opposed to usage in single tooth replacement situations. Dental implants are associated with a high degree of success and are considered a 'Permanent' solution. It should be noted that no artificial replacement currently exists without some form of limitation. The biggest drawback with long-term usage of dental implants is their susceptibility to biomechanical failure and high risk of infection. The latter situation is precarious since the structure and topography of dental implants are optimal for the commencement and perpetuation of infections. Peri-mucositis and peri-implantitis are inflammatory conditions around dental implants that can result in loss of supporting bone and failure in osseointegration. Microorganisms accumulating around dental implants can result in these inflammatory conditions in a similar manner to Gingivitis and Periodontitis around natural teeth. Peri-implantitis can progress at a faster rate around implants relative to natural teeth due to the laxity of the epithelial seal around the implant. The underlying bony tissues are, therefore, more exposed to the microflora present in the oral cavity than an intact tooth which is firmly sealed by gingival fibres and hemidesmosomal attachments.

5.1.1 What Are Biofilms?

Microbial colonisation and infective conditions cannot emerge spontaneously with just the presence of microorganisms. The human body is constantly exposed to millions of microorganisms at every minute. The major contributor to the initiation of any infection is the presence of a biofilm. Biofilms are microbial-derived sessile communities that provide a polymeric matrix or substratum for the interaction of microbes and the production of endotoxins detrimental to host tissue. Biofilms can form on any surface exposed to or in direct contact with a moist environment. Biofilms can form on tooth surfaces, catheters, implants, suction tubes, water lines and so forth [1, 2].

V. Sivaswamy (✉)
Department of Prosthodontics and Implantology, Saveetha Dental College and Hospitals, Chennai, Tamil Nadu, India

P. Neelakantan
Faculty of Dentistry, The University of Hong Kong, Hong Kong, Hong Kong
e-mail: prasanna@hku.hk

P. Neelakantan, A. Princy Solomon (eds.), *Dental Implants and Oral Microbiome Dysbiosis*,
https://doi.org/10.1007/978-3-030-99014-5_5

5.1.2 Biofilm Formation on Dental Tissue

The mechanism of biofilm formation begins with the formation of a sticky layer on the tooth surface known as the Pellicle. The pellicle is an acellular, proteinaceous film formed by the adsorption of salivary proteins on the surfaces of teeth. The pellicle is formed in a matter of seconds after the cleansing of teeth. Bacterial cells colonise on the pellicle within 4 h of its formation. Carbohydrate-binding proteins known as Lectins present on the bacterial cell surface aid in binding to carbohydrate-containing receptors on other cells. This results in cell-to-cell adhesion, known as Coaggregation, and creates multilayered clusters. The earliest colonisers are of the streptococci species (*S. sanguis*, *S. mitis* and *S. oralis*). These early colonisers are nourished by the salivary protein in supragingival biofilms and the crevicular exudate in subgingival biofilms. These organisms prepare a favourable environment for more virulent organisms such as the actinomyces species and streptococcus mutans to colonise the biofilm eventually. After a period of 2–14 days, the streptococcus-dominated population changes to an actinomyces-dominated plaque. This phenomenon is termed as Microbial succession and results in a highly diverse microbial population with increasing levels of gram-negative anaerobic, filamentous species. At this stage, the plaque or biofilm is termed mature and causes gingivitis which, if untreated, progresses to periodontitis [1–4].

5.1.3 Biofilm Formation on Implants

Biofilms on implants form the same way as described for natural teeth (Fig. 5.1). The organisms that contribute to peri-implantitis are of the *Porphyromonas*, *Prevotella*, *Capnocytophaga* and the *Fusobacterium* species [5]. These organisms produce collagenase, hyaluronidase and chondroitin sulphates, which result in the destruction of supporting tissue around the implant [2, 3, 6, 7].

Refreshing the statement made earlier, biofilms are formed on surfaces exposed to moist environments. The question then arises on how a biofilm could form on an implant surface. Dental implants are stored in a dry inert vial and are immediately embedded into bone upon removal from the vial. Once drilled into the bone, the implant is closed with a cover screw till osseointegration is complete. Oxide film is formed on the implant surface immediately upon exposure to the environment and this film renders the implant completely inert and passive. Biofilm forms on the implant once it is exposed to the oral environment during the restorative phase. The implant is exposed and fitted with an abutment which, in turn, secures the crown. The collar of the implant which is exposed to the oral cavity and the abutment-fixture interface are the primary nidus of biofilm formation. Some implant manufacturers implement a roughened collar in their implant platforms to ensure crestal bone formation and tight mucosal integration. Rough surfaces facilitate rapid biofilm formation and increase the risk of microbial colonisation. Surface free energy (SFE) is another parameter that plays a major role in predicting the formation of biofilms. Any material with a high SFE increases the risk of biofilm formation on the surface. Wettability of the material is another factor to be considered when implant biofilms are to be managed, with hydrophobic surfaces observed to be prone to biofilm formation [1, 2, 7, 8].

5.2 Biofilm Management Strategies

Preventing the formation of a salivary pellicle and subsequent biofilm, while ideal, is an unrealistic strategy. The pellicle layer will always be formed since the intraoral structures are submerged in saliva. Subsequently, microbial colonisation will occur when pellicle formation takes place. Therefore, the practical method of biofilm management will be to use materials that enable easy removal of biofilm without any damage to the surface and/or render the materials bacteriostatic or bactericidal. A combination of both

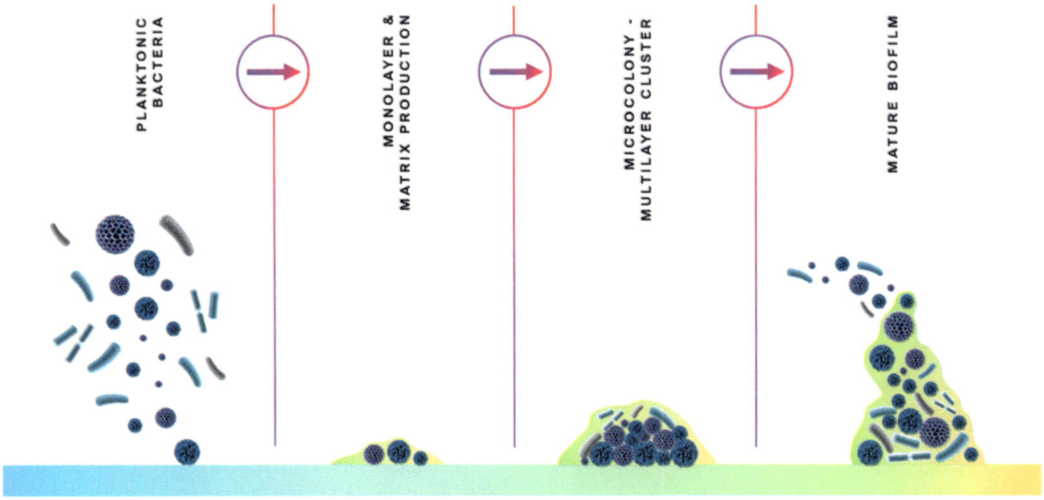

Fig. 5.1 Steps in biofilm formation

strategies may be required since a completely smooth surface is currently not available for dental applications nor an antimicrobial approach that has universal action against all spectra of microbes in the biofilm [5, 8–10].

Biofilm management can be broadly grouped into two categories—Surface Modification and Surface Coatings. Surface modification refers to the design and structural change of a material. Surface coating refers to the apposition of an auxiliary layer for various effects on existing material. Dental implants, however, are currently surface treated using a combination of both modification and coating. Therefore, the methods of biofilm management will be described below in a linear fashion without categorisation (Fig. 5.2).

Dental implant fixtures are made of Titanium alloy and a few manufacturers offer Zirconia implants. This chapter will list biofilm management strategies for these two implant materials.

5.2.1 Polymer Tethering

There have been many attempts to anchor polymer on titanium substrates to confer antimicrobial properties to implant surfaces. Physical adsorption and chemical covalent conjugation techniques are used to bond polymer molecules to titanium.

PolyNaSS (Poly-Sodium Styrene Sulfonate) is applied on the implant surface by treatment of titanium with a mixture of sulfuric acid and hydrogen peroxide followed by immersion in sodium styrene sulfonate monomer under ultraviolet (UV) irradiation. The resulting polyNaSS complex was observed to be highly bioactive and hydrophilic and inhibited *S. aureus* by 70% when compared with non-treated titanium surfaces [11].

PolyNIPAM (Poly *N*-Isopropylacrylamide) is a thermo-responsive polymer which exhibits a lower critical solubility temperature (LCST) in water at 32 °C. Below LCST, the material is hydrophilic while a rise in temperature above LCST renders the material hydrophobic. Lee et al. coated titanium surfaces with polyNIPAM and observed a reduction in bacterial adhesion when temperatures decreased below LCST [12].

Schaer et al. utilised a hydrophobic polycation (*N*,*N*-dodecyl, methyl polyethyleneimine) on titanium and observed that biofilm formation was inhibited [13].

PEG (Polyethylene glycol) chains are resistant to protein adsorption since they act as a barrier created by structured water and steric repulsion. PEG chains are immobilised on titanium via self-assembly, silanisation, physisorption and plasma polymerisation. These coatings have proven effective against *S. sanguinis* and *L.*

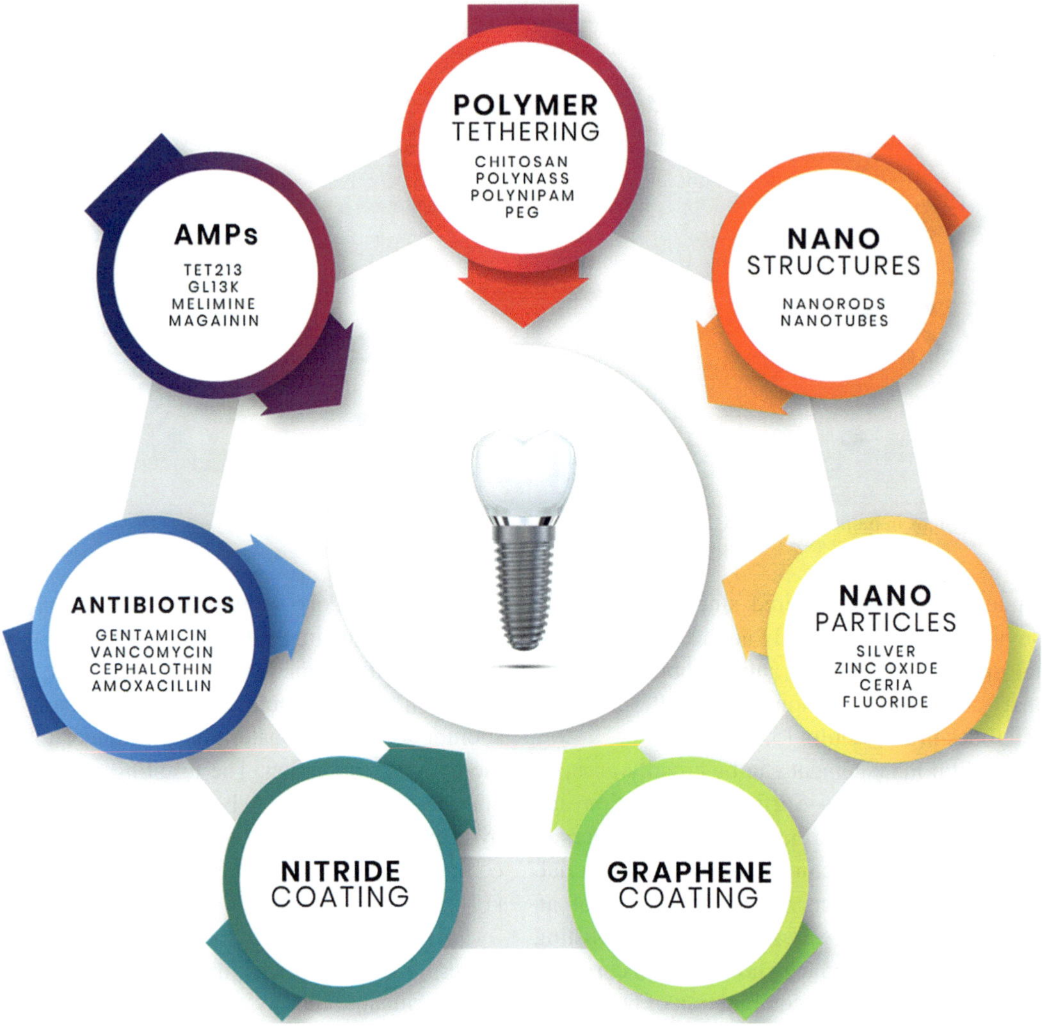
POLYMER
TETHERING
CHITOSAN
POLYNASS
POLYNIPAM
PEG
NANO
STRUCTURES
NANORODS
NANOTUBES
NANO
PARTICLES
SILVER
ZINC OXIDE
CERIA
FLUORIDE
GRAPHENE
COATING
NITRIDE
COATING
ANTIBIOTICS
GENTAMICIN
VANCOMYCIN
CEPHALOTHIN
AMOXACILLIN
AMPs
TET213
GL13K
MELIMINE
MAGAININ

Fig. 5.2 Summary of antibiofilm strategies for dental implants

salivarious by reducing their adhesion to the material surface [14, 15].

5.2.2 Chitosan

Chitosan is a cationic polysaccharide and was discovered by Rouget in 1859. It is a copolymer comprised of 2-amino-2-deoxyglucose and 2-acetylamino-2-deoxyglucose-D-glucoside. It can be manufactured synthetically or derived from natural chitin. Rouget treated chitin with hot potassium hydroxide and observed that deacetylation of chitin produces chitosan. It is rich in amino groups and is highly soluble as well as biocompatible. It has excellent biodegradability and can be reduced to non-toxic residue by lysozyme. It has been found to be non-antigenic, anti-inflammatory and hemostatic. These properties have led to the implementation of chitosan in hemostatic gels, paste, dressings and drug delivery systems for local dosing [16–20].

Chitosan has been observed to possess excellent metal binding and antimicrobial properties. In vitro studies coating chitosan on titanium surfaces demonstrated enhanced fibroblast cell attachment and proliferation on titanium as well as inhibition of *Porphyromonas gingivalis*. Low molecular weight chitosan could breach bacterial cell walls and result in bacterial elimination. High levels of osteoblast cell growth and bone formation have also been observed in laboratory studies. Chitosan could be employed as a gene carrier to deliver transcription factor for promoting bone formation. Targeted delivery of bone-inducing agents could result in predictable implant therapy in osteoporotic conditions [18, 21–24].

Chitosan nanoparticles can be prepared using various methods, with the most common method being *Ionic Gelation*. Chitosan is dissolved in acetic acid solution with a tinge of sodium hydroxide to adjust pH. TPP (tripolyphosphate) is added to the aqueous chitosan as a cross-linking agent and magnetically stirred under room temperature to obtain chitosan nanoparticles. This method produces nanoparticles in the 90 nm range and is widely used as drug delivery systems [16, 25].

Solvent evaporation is another method wherein the chitosan solution is made into an emulsion and polymer solvent is added. The solvent evaporates and precipitates into nanospheres. A Tris buffer with ethanol is used to keep the pH stable and the mixture is stirred magnetically for 30 min. The solvent is removed, and the nanoparticle yield is obtained. Studies using this method have produced blends of chitosan with silver nanoparticles with claims of potent antimicrobial action [25, 26].

Microemulsion method produces chitosan nanoparticles by forming reverse micelles that contain a large volume of organic solvents with water cores. This results in droplets of material in the nanoscale range. This method is time-consuming, expensive and employs a large volume of solvents [25].

Self-assembly involves the production of nanoparticles without any organic solvents or cross-linking agents. Nanoparticles are formed by mixing positive chitosan polysaccharides and negative phospholipids. The two components complex together via electrostatic interaction and produce nanoparticles with a high encapsulation efficiency [25].

5.2.3 Functionalisation with Anchor Molecules

Anchor molecules are grafted to metallic substrates to impart bioactive functionalisation. Anchors that have been tested for functionalisation include silane, catechol and phosphate anchors.

Silane anchorage involves organofunctional alkoxysilane molecules that react with hydroxyl groups on material surface. Antimicrobial peptides are attached with these anchor molecules to render titanium surfaces bacteriostatic. Melimine, a synthetic antimicrobial peptide, possessing broad-spectrum action against bacteria and fungi, has been tethered to titanium modified with silane anchors into a maleimide functionalised surface. Melimine was observed to reduce adhesion of *Pseudomonas aeruginosa* and *S. aureus* on titanium surfaces. Commercial antibiotics such as vancomycin and caspofungin have also been grafted to titanium surfaces and observed to reduce adhesion of *S. aureus* and *C. albicans* biofilms by 99% compared to non-grafted titanium surfaces [27, 28].

Catechol anchors have been used to tether PolyNaSS to titanium surfaces for a bacteriostatic effect. The dopamine-linked PolyNaSS resulted in inhibition of *S. aureus* up to 65%, depending on the molecular weight of the molecule, with bigger polymers exhibiting higher antibacterial effect. Carboxymethyl chitosan and antimicrobial peptide Magainin has also been grafted to titanium using dopamine, with each group individually reducing bacterial counts significantly. Polydopamine and silver coating using micro arc oxidation and immersion have shown effective retardation of microbial growth and colonisation [29, 30].

Silane and catechol anchors, however, are unstable in aqueous environments at physiologic pH and may not be a feasible option in routine clinical conditions, Phosphate anchors lack this limitation and offer stable tethering for biomedical applications. Myo-inositol hexaphosphate linked to titanium substrates demonstrated reduced adhesion of *S. sanguinis*. Other examples of phosphate-linked antimicrobial grafts include 4-vinylpryridine with vinylbenzylphosphonate and 4-vinyl *N*-hexylpyridinium bromide (HBVP) [31].

5.2.4 Nanostructures

Nanotechnology deals with the design, characterisation and application of structures in the nanometre scale. Nanostructured surfaces are of great interest in dental implantology since they have been observed to confer enhanced biologic integration as well as antimicrobial properties on titanium. It was observed that TiO_2 nanotubes display antibacterial properties. A combination of heat treatment and nanostructured patterning through anodisation has been observed to reduce the number of dead and live bacterial cells in laboratory studies. Anatase surfaces of titanium were also found to be antimicrobial when compared with rutile surfaces. Lin *et al.* loaded titanium nanotubes with gentamicin using the lyophilisation method and vacuum drying and reported strong antibacterial action with an extended drug release time [32, 33].

5.2.5 Nanoparticles

Nanoparticles are ultrafine particles with dimensions ranging from 1 to 100 nm. Nanoparticles have been applied to titanium surfaces in laboratory studies to enhance hard and soft tissue integration. Current surface coating methods for nanoparticles include dip-coating, self-assembly, spin coating, freeze thaw, plasma spray, electrospinning, magnetron sputtering, anodisation, pulsed electrodeposition, nano-spray drying and covalent binding [34].

5.2.5.1 Silver Nanoparticles

Silver is a known antibacterial agent and has been used to treat bacterial infections since time immemorial in various forms, such as metallic silver, silver nitrate and silver sulfadiazine. Silver nanoparticles contain 100–15,000 atoms with diameters smaller than 100 nm. They possess a large surface-to-volume ratio and excellent antimicrobial activity leading to their incorporation into acrylic resins for dentures, coatings in titanium dental implants, irrigation and obturation in endodontic therapy and membranes for periodontal tissue regeneration. Silver nanoparticles continually release silver ions that adhere to the bacterial cell walls and alter their permeability. Silver ions disrupt respiratory enzymes, interrupt adenosine triphosphate production and generate reactive oxygen species (ROS). ROS can disrupt cell membrane and deoxyribonucleic acid (DNA) expression. Furthermore, silver ions can also denature ribosomes and inhibit protein synthesis. The antibacterial effect of silver is dependent on the dissolution of the nanoparticle, particle size and shape. Smaller sized particles are observed to release more silver ions due to their larger surface area. The presence of organic and inorganic components can also influence the availability of silver ions by forming complexes with silver nanoparticles. Gram-negative bacteria are more susceptible since the cell wall is narrower than gram-positive species. Thicker biofilms, however, might prevent the silver ions from reaching the bacterial colonies harbouring within, thereby reducing the antibacterial effect of silver. Silver nanoparticles smaller than 50 nm are necessary to predictably enter the biofilm and exert action on the bacterial cell wall. Modifying implant surfaces with doped silver nanoparticles has been under investigation over an extended duration. However, there are no commercial implants with embedded or coated silver nanoparticles available for routine clinical usage. The results of laboratory studies appear to be promising, with silver nanoparticles demonstrating strong bactericidal action against *S. aureus* and *P. aeruginosa* while exhibiting low cytotoxicity on osteoblastic cells. One major area of investigation is the long-term assessment of silver nanoparticles on human cells. The mechanism of action for silver particles described earlier is non-discriminatory in nature. The silver particles could induce oxidative stress and interfere with ATP production in human cells. There are also concerns about the detection of silver in the liver and spleen after systemic doses. Another concern is that the size of the particles is small enough to breach the blood-brain barrier. This could result in unforeseen morbidities for patients constantly exposed to silver nanoparticles [28, 35–38].

5.2.5.2 Zinc Oxide Nanoparticles

ZnO nanoparticles have exhibited antibacterial activity against both gram-positive and -negative organisms via the generation of reactive oxygen species as well as the accumulation of particles on the bacterial cell surface. ZnO nanoparticles have been combined with hydroxyapatite to form a coating over titanium surfaces. A 75/25% ratio of ZnO and HA displayed considerable antimicrobial action along with minimal toxicity on MG63 cells [39–41].

5.2.5.3 Copper Oxide Nanoparticles

Copper nanoparticles have an antibacterial action similar to that of zinc with a major drawback of rapid oxidation on exposure to air. CuO nanoparticles have been coated on dental implant surfaces and observed to exhibit inhibitory zones, which retarded the growth of test bacteria [41, 42].

5.2.5.4 Quercitrin Nanoparticles

Quercitrin is a glycoside derivative of the flavonoid Quercetin and Rhamnose, with a high potential to improve soft tissue healing. In vitro testing by Gomez-Florit *et al.* revealed potent anti-inflammatory action with increased fibroblast attachment, increased collagen mRNA levels and decreased matrix metalloproteinase and prostaglandin E2 [43, 44].

5.2.5.5 Chlorhexidine Nanoparticles

2% Chlorhexidine (CHX) is recommended for the treatment of mucositis and peri-implantitis in conjunction with mechanical debridement. CHX achieves biofilm reduction depending on concentration with 2% concentration being the optimal level for 96–99% reduction [45]. Barbour et al. studied the effect of CHX immersion on anatase and rutile titanium surfaces and found a reduction in bacterial coverage by 80% in the anatase surfaces [46]. Chlorhexidine coatings are employed in the internal chamber of PIXIT implants to curb the incidence of biofilm formation along the fixture-abutment interface [47].

5.2.5.6 Titanium Dioxide Nanoparticles

TiO_2 nanoparticles can be coated on titanium surfaces using a sol-gel method to increase osteoblast cell proliferation resulting in improved implant stability. TiO_2 can also be applied using the anodic oxidation method which is routinely used to increase the thickness of the oxide layer. In vitro studies have revealed significantly enhanced cell attachment, proliferation and osteogenic differentiation [38, 48].

5.2.5.7 Nanocrystalline Diamond

Nanocrystalline diamond coating around titanium surfaces exhibits high corrosion resistance and biologic compatibility. The coating forms a protective barrier around the implant preventing the release of metallic ions into the body. Adequate bone-implant contact (BIC) percentage has been observed by Metzler *et al.* with diamond coatings around Ti-6Al-4V alloys [49].

5.2.5.8 Ceria Nanoparticles

Ceria nanoparticles in the form of nano-rods, nano-cubes and nano-octahedron around titanium surface were found to exhibit strong antibacterial and anti-inflammatory action. Ceria coating is advantageous over other metallic nanoparticles since it is an ROS scavenger. Ag and ZnO nanoparticles generate ROS radicals which may harm human tissue through oxidative stress indiscriminately and this dose-dependent cytotoxicity limits their application. Ceria can be coated using plasma spray, spin coating and magnetron sputtering methods. The antibacterial action of ceria is through electrostatic attraction between the positively charged CeO_2 and the negatively charged cell wall and/or their interaction with sulfhydryl groups in the cell surface proteins. CeO_2 is capable of switching between valence states and can exist as Ce^{3+} and Ce^{4+} ions. Ce^{3+} ions are superoxide mimetic whereas Ce^{4+} ions are catalase mimetic. The initial concentration of Ce^{3+} ions results in antibacterial action with the production of H_2O_2, a destructive oxygen species which is then converted to O_2 and H_2O by the catalase mimetic action of Ce^{4+}, thereby reducing the risk of damage to non-microbial host cells [50, 51].

5.2.6 Antimicrobial Peptides

Antimicrobial peptides (AMPs) are a group of peptide molecules also known as Host Defence Peptides (HDPs) that are part of the innate immune system of living organisms. AMPs display a wide range of activities being antiviral, antibacterial, antiparasitic and antifungal. They can be derived from human as well as animal sources. Human-derived peptides are advantageous over antibiotics since they are biocompatible, display low host cytotoxicity and possess broad spectral activity. Peptides can be tethered to titanium to confer an antimicrobial effect to inhibit biofilm formation. Tet213, a cationic peptide, bound to titanium has demonstrated bactericidal action on *S. aureus* and *P. aeruginosa* [52].

One major drawback with most AMPs is their vulnerability to protease activity. Gorr *et al.* (2012), developed an AMP derived from parotid secretory protein (BPIFA2), which displays potent anti-inflammatory and antibacterial action. This peptide has been titled GL13K and is highly resistant to protease activity as well as mechanical challenges. GL13K bound to titanium displayed bactericidal action against *P. gingivalis*, *P. aeruginosa* and *Strep. gordonii* [53–56].

5.2.7 Ion Implanted Surfaces

Fluorine, Zinc, Calcium, Chlorine, Iodine, Copper, Cerium and Selenium ions have been implanted to titanium surfaces individually in various laboratory studies. Anodic oxidation is used to embed these ions on the substrate. These ions confer bactericidal action upon dissolution into surrounding tissues and undergo hydroxylation into reaction species such as HOCL, TiOH and O^{2-} (Superoxide). Reactive species oxidise bacterial cell membranes and increase cell permeability resulting in cell death [50]. Shirai *et al.* demonstrated the effectiveness of iodine implanted titanium fixtures in patients with successful clinical outcomes [57–61]. The other ion implantations have only been tested in vitro and clinical evidence is yet to be produced.

5.2.8 Photocatalytic Titanium

TiO_2 (Titanium dioxide) is typically non-toxic and photoactive under aerobic conditions. Ultraviolet A radiation (UVA) with wavelengths between 315 and 380 nm for 120 min imparts photo-functionalisation of TiO_2 and removes hydrocarbon contamination. UVA irradiation results in a super hydrophilic surface (contact angle less than 20°), which oxidises adsorbed organic impurities and produces reactive oxygen species, thereby rendering the titanium surface highly antimicrobial. Hydroxyl radicals (HO^-) and H_2O_2 are produced that can destroy the bacterial cell membrane [62–66].

5.2.9 Antibiotics

Antibiotic coatings of gentamicin, vancomycin, cephalothin, carbenicillin, amoxicillin and tobramycin have been tested on implant surfaces with initially strong bactericidal action gradually losing potency due to elution of the antibiotic [12, 67–71]. Local and systemic toxicity is another parameter that is yet to be investigated in a clinical scenario.

5.2.10 Graphene

Graphene is a one-dimensional single atom thick layer of carbon atoms connected in a hexagonal configuration. Dry and wet transfer techniques have been used to coat graphene on titanium surfaces. Thin films of graphene with silver nanoparticles have been observed to inhibit *S. mutans* and *P. gingivalis* with cell viability inversely proportional to the concentration of graphene and silver [39, 72–74].

5.2.11 Nitride Coatings

Titanium nitride offers excellent chemical stability, corrosion resistance and enhanced hardness. The characteristic golden colour of titanium nitride aids in the camouflage of the metallic fixture components under gingival tissue, leading to better aesthetics. Nitride coatings have exhibited antibacterial effect against *S. mutans* [75–77].

5.3 Coating Methods

5.3.1 Anodic Oxidation

Anodic oxidation or anodisation is an electrochemical method where the metal substrate is the anode immersed in an electrolyte solution such as sulfuric acid, hydrogen peroxide and phosphoric acid along with a cathode and subjected to electrical discharges. The discharge produces oxygen that bonds with the anode thereby oxidising it and the cathode undergoes a reduction reaction. Anodisation is commonly used in coating industries to provide a thick oxide layer on metal substrates for various effects. Dental implants are subjected to anodisation to provide a thick TiO_2 oxide layer to aid in osseointegration and faster cellular proliferation [33, 78, 79].

5.3.2 Plasma Spray

Plasma spray consists of deposition of fine droplets in the molten or semi-molten state to form a coating. The coating material is rapidly heated by accelerating it through a plasma flame (10,000–30,000 K). The heated material melts down as it passes through the flame and lands on the substrate surface where it hardens on cooling to form a coating [80].

5.3.3 Plasma Immersion Ion Implantation

PIII, also known as pulsed plasma doping, is a process where ions accelerated through plasma are retrieved using a high voltage pulsed DC and redirecting these ions onto a substrate with a semiconductor wafer to implant with doping agents. The plasma is generated in a specially designed vacuum chamber using glow discharge or metal vapour arc methods [81].

5.3.4 Physical Vapour Deposition

A method of coating where solid metal is vapourised in a vacuum environment and deposited on substrate materials. Titanium nitride coatings can be made using physical vapour deposition. Physical vapour deposition can also be performed using magnetron sputtering wherein a gold/palladium conductive coating is required to prevent charging of a specimen [82].

5.3.5 Chemical Vapour Deposition

Chemical vapour deposition (CVD) is a coating technique in which thin films are formed on a heated substrate via a chemical reaction of gaseous precursors. Carbon nanotubes and graphene coatings are achieved using the CVD method [83].

5.3.6 Sol-Gel Method

Sol-gel is a process where suspension of monomers in a liquid medium results in a colloidal solution (Sol) which undergoes hydrolysis and condensation polymerisation to form the semisolid gel. The gel is then coated to the substrate where it dries into a thin hard film [28].

5.4 Limitations of Current Evidence

It should be noted that the methods described earlier are bound by the limitations of laboratory studies. Majority of these methods have tested antibacterial efficacy using a monoculture model under static growth conditions. Dental implants are in constant contact with physiologic fluids and are also under biomechanical load. A single species or a single host protein does not accurately reflect the complex interactions observed in the oral environment. Cytotoxicity and biocompatibility data are also lacking for most of these methods, which precludes progression to clinical trials.

Dental implants are drilled into bone for stable anchorage to initiate the process of osseointegration. Implant placement into the prepared osteotomy site involves tight threading, which may disrupt the surface coatings or modifications. The status of these coatings and characterisation needs to be evaluated post-surgically to verify their integrity and biologic effect.

5.5 Clinical Application

A clinically relevant yet economical method of applying these techniques would be to limit the coating and/or modification to the most biofilm-prone areas of the target material (i.e. dental implant). The implant-abutment interface is at high risk for biofilm formation since this region is enveloped by the gingival soft tissue. This soft tissue cuff is simply braced against the implant and abutment surface as opposed to a tight integration by gingival fibres as observed in natural dentition. In a nutshell, the areas of the implant in direct contact with the surrounding soft tissue are the most vulnerable to microbial colonisation due to a combination of constant salivary and crevicular fluid contact and the surface roughness of the material (Fig. 5.3). The logical step, then, is to render the implant platform and abutment interface inert to biofilm formation using the above-mentioned methods. Preventing biofilm formation in these areas would prevent microbial colonisation and in turn, reduce the incidence of inflammatory conditions such as peri-implant mucositis and peri-implantitis.

Conflict of Interest The authors are not affiliated to any of the commercial manufacturers or firms mentioned in this chapter or are sponsored, in any way, for the active promotion or marketing of any product described in the chapter.

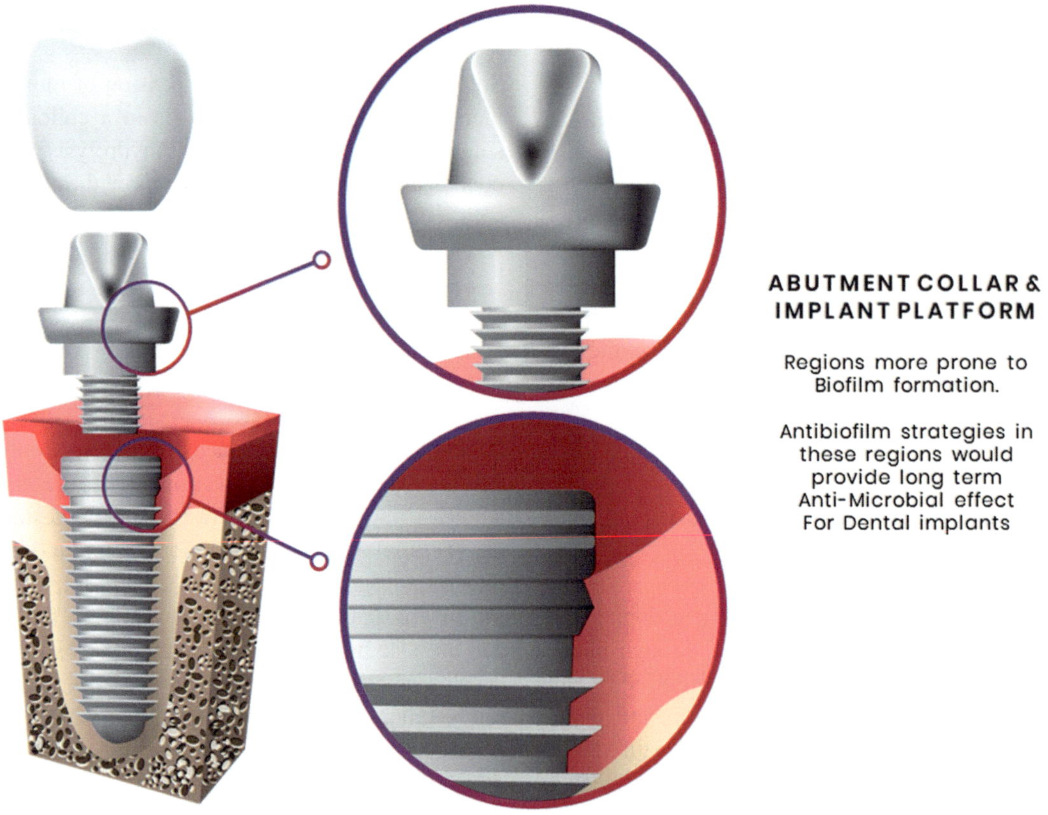

Fig. 5.3 Biofilm-prone areas in dental implants

References

1. Subramani K, Jung RE, Molenberg A, Hammerle CHF. Biofilm on dental implants: a review of the literature. Int J Oral Maxillofac Implants. 2009;24(4):616–26.
2. Lee A, Wang H-L. Biofilm related to dental implants. Implant Dent. 2010;19(5):387–93.
3. Busscher HJ, Rinastiti M, Siswomihardjo W, van der Mei HC. Biofilm formation on dental restorative and implant materials. J Dent Res. 2010;89(7):657–65.
4. Bordin D, Cavalcanti IMG, Jardim Pimentel M, Fortulan CA, Sotto-Maior BS, Del Bel Cury AA, et al. Biofilm and saliva affect the biomechanical behavior of dental implants. J Biomech. 2015;48(6):997–1002.
5. Lafaurie GI, Sabogal MA, Castillo DM, Rincón MV, Gómez LA, Lesmes YA, et al. Microbiome and microbial biofilm profiles of peri-implantitis: a systematic review. J Periodontol. 2017;88(10):1066–89.
6. Esfahanizadeh N, Mirmalek SP, Bahador A, Daneshparvar H, Akhoundi N, Pourhajibagher M. Formation of biofilm on various implant abutment materials. Gen Dent. 2018;66(5):39–44.
7. Valen H, Scheie AA. Biofilms and their properties. Eur J Oral Sci. 2018;126(Suppl 1):13–8.
8. Daubert DM, Weinstein BF. Biofilm as a risk factor in implant treatment. Periodontol 2000. 2019;81(1):29–40.
9. Larsen T, Fiehn N-E. Dental biofilm infections—an update. APMIS Acta Pathol Microbiol Immunol Scand. 2017;125(4):376–84.
10. Marsh PD, Zaura E. Dental biofilm: ecological interactions in health and disease. J Clin Periodontol. 2017;44(Suppl 18):S12–22.
11. Alcheikh A, Pavon-Djavid G, Helary G, Petite H, Migonney V, Anagnostou F. PolyNaSS grafting on titanium surfaces enhances osteoblast differentiation and inhibits Staphylococcus aureus adhesion. J Mater Sci Mater Med. 2013;24(7):1745–54.
12. Teratanatorn P, Hoskins R, Swift T, Douglas CWI, Shepherd J, Rimmer S. Binding of bacteria to poly(N-isopropylacrylamide) modified with vancomycin: comparison of behavior of linear and highly branched polymers. Biomacromolecules. 2017;18(9):2887–99.
13. Schaer TP, Stewart S, Hsu BB, Klibanov AM. Hydrophobic polycationic coatings that inhibit biofilms and support bone healing during infection. Biomaterials. 2012;33(5):1245–54.
14. Buxadera-Palomero J, Calvo C, Torrent-Camarero S, Gil FJ, Mas-Moruno C, Canal C, et al. Biofunctional polyethylene glycol coatings on titanium: an in vitro-based comparison of functionalization methods. Colloids Surf B Biointerfaces. 2017;152:367–75.
15. Buxadera-Palomero J, Canal C, Torrent-Camarero S, Garrido B, Javier Gil F, Rodríguez D. Antifouling coatings for dental implants: polyethylene glycol-like coatings on titanium by plasma polymerization. Biointerphases. 2015;10(2):029505.
16. Bumgardner JD, Wiser R, Gerard PD, Bergin P, Chestnutt B, Marin M, et al. Chitosan: potential use as a bioactive coating for orthopaedic and craniofacial/dental implants. J Biomater Sci Polym Ed. 2003;14(5):423–38.
17. Lin M-H, Wang Y-H, Kuo C-H, Ou S-F, Huang P-Z, Song T-Y, et al. Hybrid ZnO/chitosan antimicrobial coatings with enhanced mechanical and bioactive properties for titanium implants. Carbohydr Polym. 2021;257:117639.
18. Divakar DD, Jastaniyah NT, Altamimi HG, Alnakhli YO, et al. Enhanced antimicrobial activity of naturally derived bioactive molecule chitosan conjugated silver nanoparticle against dental implant pathogens. Int J Biol Macromol. 2018;108:790–7.
19. Cicciù M, Fiorillo L, Cervino G. Chitosan use in dentistry: a systematic review of recent clinical studies. Mar Drugs. 2019;17(7):E417.
20. Lestari W, Yusry WNAW, Haris MS, Jaswir I, Idrus E. A glimpse on the function of chitosan as a dental hemostatic agent. Jpn Dent Sci Rev. 2020;56(1):147–54.
21. Lv H, Chen Z, Yang X, Cen L, Zhang X, Gao P. Layer-by-layer self-assembly of minocycline-loaded chitosan/alginate multilayer on titanium substrates to inhibit biofilm formation. J Dent. 2014;42(11):1464–72.
22. Correa DS, Tayalia P, Cosendey G, dos Santos DS, Aroca RF, Mazur E, et al. Two-photon polymerization for fabricating structures containing the biopolymer chitosan. J Nanosci Nanotechnol. 2009;9(10):5845–9.
23. Zhang T, Zhang X, Mao M, Li J, Wei T, Sun H. Chitosan/hydroxyapatite composite coatings on porous Ti6Al4V titanium implants: in vitro and in vivo studies. J Periodontal Implant Sci. 2020;50(6):392–405.
24. Aguilar A, Zein N, Harmouch E, Hafdi B, Bornert F, Offner D, et al. Application of chitosan in bone and dental engineering. Mol Basel Switz. 2019;24(16):E3009.
25. Zhang C, Hui D, Du C, Sun H, Peng W, Pu X, et al. Preparation and application of chitosan biomaterials in dentistry. Int J Biol Macromol. 2021;167:1198–210.
26. Fakhri E, Eslami H, Maroufi P, Pakdel F, Taghizadeh S, Ganbarov K, et al. Chitosan biomaterials application in dentistry. Int J Biol Macromol. 2020;162:956–74.
27. Godoy-Gallardo M, Guillem-Marti J, Sevilla P, Manero JM, Gil FJ, Rodriguez D. Anhydride-functional silane immobilized onto titanium surfaces induces osteoblast cell differentiation and reduces bacterial adhesion and biofilm formation. Mater Sci Eng C Mater Biol Appl. 2016;59:524–32.
28. Babapour A, Yang B, Bahang S, Cao W. Low-temperature sol-gel-derived nanosilver-embedded silane coating as biofilm inhibitor. Nanotechnology. 2011;22(15):155602.
29. Zhang W, Wang S, Ge S, Chen J, Ji P. The relationship between substrate morphology and biological performances of nano-silver-loaded dopamine coatings on titanium surfaces. R Soc Open Sci. 2018;5(4):172310.

30. Singh I, Dhawan G, Gupta S, Kumar P. Recent advances in a polydopamine-mediated antimicrobial adhesion system. Front Microbiol. 2020;11:607099.
31. Pawar AA, Saada G, Cooperstein I, Larush L, Jackman JA, Tabaei SR, et al. High-performance 3D printing of hydrogels by water-dispersible photoinitiator nanoparticles. Sci Adv. 2016;2(4):e1501381.
32. Grenho L, Salgado CL, Fernandes MH, Monteiro FJ, Ferraz MP. Antibacterial activity and biocompatibility of three-dimensional nanostructured porous granules of hydroxyapatite and zinc oxide nanoparticles—an in vitro and in vivo study. Nanotechnology. 2015;26(31):315101.
33. Lee J, Park S, Kang S, Park C, Yun K. Bonding evaluation between nanotube by anodic oxidation and machined dental titanium implant in beagle dog. J Nanosci Nanotechnol. 2019;19(2):912–4.
34. Gulati K, Ivanovski S. Dental implants modified with drug releasing titania nanotubes: therapeutic potential and developmental challenges. Expert Opin Drug Deliv. 2017;14(8):1009–24.
35. Noronha VT, Paula AJ, Durán G, Galembeck A, Cogo-Müller K, Franz-Montan M, et al. Silver nanoparticles in dentistry. Dent Mater Off Publ Acad Dent Mater. 2017;33(10):1110–26.
36. Qin H, Cao H, Zhao Y, Zhu C, Cheng T, Wang Q, et al. In vitro and in vivo anti-biofilm effects of silver nanoparticles immobilized on titanium. Biomaterials. 2014;35(33):9114–25.
37. Piszczek P, Lewandowska Ż, Radtke A, Jędrzejewski T, Kozak W, Sadowska B, et al. Biocompatibility of titania nanotube coatings enriched with silver nanograins by chemical vapor deposition. Nanomater Basel Switz. 2017;7(9):E274.
38. Gunputh UF, Le H, Lawton K, Besinis A, Tredwin C, Handy RD. Antibacterial properties of silver nanoparticles grown in situ and anchored to titanium dioxide nanotubes on titanium implant against Staphylococcus aureus. Nanotoxicology. 2020;14(1):97–110.
39. Kulshrestha S, Khan S, Meena R, Singh BR, Khan AU. A graphene/zinc oxide nanocomposite film protects dental implant surfaces against cariogenic Streptococcus mutans. Biofouling. 2014;30(10):1281–94.
40. Mahamuni-Badiger PP, Patil PM, Badiger MV, Patel PR, Thorat-Gadgil BS, Pandit A, et al. Biofilm formation to inhibition: role of zinc oxide-based nanoparticles. Mater Sci Eng C Mater Biol Appl. 2020;108:110319.
41. Vergara-Llanos D, Koning T, Pavicic MF, Bello-Toledo H, Díaz-Gómez A, Jaramillo A, et al. Antibacterial and cytotoxic evaluation of copper and zinc oxide nanoparticles as a potential disinfectant material of connections in implant provisional abutments: an in-vitro study. Arch Oral Biol. 2021;122:105031.
42. Bergemann C, Zaatreh S, Wegner K, Arndt K, Podbielski A, Bader R, et al. Copper as an alternative antimicrobial coating for implants—an in vitro study. World J Transplant. 2017;7(3):193–202.
43. Gomez-Florit M, Pacha-Olivenza MA, Fernández-Calderón MC, Córdoba A, González-Martín ML, Monjo M, et al. Quercitrin-nanocoated titanium surfaces favour gingival cells against oral bacteria. Sci Rep. 2016;6:22444.
44. Córdoba A, Manzanaro-Moreno N, Colom C, Rønold HJ, Lyngstadaas SP, Monjo M, et al. Quercitrin nanocoated implant surfaces reduce osteoclast activity in vitro and in vivo. Int J Mol Sci. 2018;19(11):E3319.
45. Wood NJ, Jenkinson HF, Davis SA, Mann S, O'Sullivan DJ, Barbour ME. Chlorhexidine hexametaphosphate nanoparticles as a novel antimicrobial coating for dental implants. J Mater Sci Mater Med. 2015;26(6):201.
46. Barbour ME, Gandhi N, el-Turki A, O'Sullivan DJ, Jagger DC. Differential adhesion of Streptococcus gordonii to anatase and rutile titanium dioxide surfaces with and without functionalization with chlorhexidine. J Biomed Mater Res A. 2009;90(4):993–8.
47. Carinci F, Lauritano D, Bignozzi CA, Pazzi D, Candotto V, Santos de Oliveira P, et al. A new strategy against peri-implantitis: antibacterial internal coating. Int J Mol Sci. 2019;20(16) E3897
48. Ribeiro AR, Gemini-Piperni S, Travassos R, Lemgruber L, Silva RC, Rossi AL, et al. Trojan-like internalization of anatase titanium dioxide nanoparticles by human osteoblast cells. Sci Rep. 2016;6:23615.
49. Metzler P, von Wilmowsky C, Stadlinger B, Zemann W, Schlegel KA, Rosiwal S, et al. Nano-crystalline diamond-coated titanium dental implants—a histomorphometric study in adult domestic pigs. J Craniomaxillofac Surg. 2013;41(6):532–8.
50. Li X, Qi M, Sun X, Weir MD, Tay FR, Oates TW, et al. Surface treatments on titanium implants via nanostructured ceria for antibacterial and anti-inflammatory capabilities. Acta Biomater. 2019;94:627–43.
51. Gagnon J, Clift MJD, Vanhecke D, Kuhn DA, Weber P, Petri-Fink A, et al. Integrating silver compounds and nanoparticles into ceria nanocontainers for antimicrobial applications. J Mater Chem B. 2015;3(9):1760–8.
52. Wang Z, Shen Y, Haapasalo M. Antibiofilm peptides against oral biofilms. J Oral Microbiol. 2017;9(1):1327308.
53. Bechinger B, Gorr S-U. Antimicrobial peptides: mechanisms of action and resistance. J Dent Res. 2017;96(3):254–60.
54. Chen X, Hirt H, Li Y, Gorr S-U, Aparicio C. Antimicrobial GL13K peptide coatings killed and ruptured the wall of Streptococcus gordonii and prevented formation and growth of biofilms. PLoS One. 2014;9(11):e111579.
55. Hirt H, Gorr S-U. Antimicrobial peptide GL13K is effective in reducing biofilms of Pseudomonas aeruginosa. Antimicrob Agents Chemother. 2013;57(10):4903–10.
56. Hirt H, Hall JW, Larson E, Gorr S-U. A D-enantiomer of the antimicrobial peptide GL13K evades antimicrobial resistance in the Gram positive bacteria

Enterococcus faecalis and Streptococcus gordonii. PLoS One. 2018;13(3):e0194900.
57. Shirai T, Tsuchiya H, Terauchi R, Tsuchida S, Mizoshiri N, Mori Y, et al. A retrospective study of antibacterial iodine-coated implants for postoperative infection. Medicine (Baltimore). 2019;98(45):e17932.
58. Shirai T, Shimizu T, Ohtani K, Zen Y, Takaya M, Tsuchiya H. Antibacterial iodine-supported titanium implants. Acta Biomater. 2011;7(4):1928–33.
59. Inoue D, Kabata T, Kajino Y, Shirai T, Tsuchiya H. Iodine-supported titanium implants have good antimicrobial attachment effects. J Orthop Sci. 2019;24(3):548–51.
60. Tsuchiya H, Shirai T, Nishida H, Murakami H, Kabata T, Yamamoto N, et al. Innovative antimicrobial coating of titanium implants with iodine. J Orthop Sci. 2012;17(5):595–604.
61. Ueoka K, Kajino Y, Kabata T, Inoue D, Yoshitani J, Ueno T, et al. The feasibility of iodine-supported processing for titanium with different surfaces. J Orthop Sci. 2020;25(6):1095–100.
62. Jia L, Qiu J, Du L, Li Z, Liu H, Ge S. TiO_2 nanorod arrays as a photocatalytic coating enhanced antifungal and antibacterial efficiency of Ti substrates. Nanomedicine. 2017;12(7):761–76.
63. Nagay BE, Dini C, Cordeiro JM, Ricomini-Filho AP, de Avila ED, Rangel EC, et al. Visible-light-induced photocatalytic and antibacterial activity of TiO_2 codoped with nitrogen and bismuth: new perspectives to control implant-biofilm-related diseases. ACS Appl Mater Interfaces. 2019;11(20):18186–202.
64. Rupp F, Haupt M, Eichler M, Doering C, Klostermann H, Scheideler L, et al. Formation and photocatalytic decomposition of a pellicle on anatase surfaces. J Dent Res. 2012;91(1):104–9.
65. Pantaroto HN, Ricomini-Filho AP, Bertolini MM, Dias da Silva JH, Azevedo Neto NF, Sukotjo C, et al. Antibacterial photocatalytic activity of different crystalline TiO_2 phases in oral multispecies biofilm. Dent Mater. 2018;34(7):e182–95.
66. Jain S, Williamson RS, Marquart M, Janorkar AV, Griggs JA, Roach MD. Photofunctionalization of anodized titanium surfaces using UVA or UVC light and its effects against Streptococcus sanguinis. J Biomed Mater Res B Appl Biomater. 2018;106(6):2284–94.
67. Bidossi A, Bottagisio M, Logoluso N, De Vecchi E. In vitro evaluation of gentamicin or vancomycin containing bone graft substitute in the prevention of orthopedic implant-related infections. Int J Mol Sci. 2020;21(23):E9250.
68. Butini ME, Cabric S, Trampuz A, Di Luca M. In vitro anti-biofilm activity of a biphasic gentamicin-loaded calcium sulfate/hydroxyapatite bone graft substitute. Colloids Surf B Biointerfaces. 2018;161:252–60.
69. Diefenbeck M, Schrader C, Gras F, Mückley T, Schmidt J, Zankovych S, et al. Gentamicin coating of plasma chemical oxidized titanium alloy prevents implant-related osteomyelitis in rats. Biomaterials. 2016;101:156–64.
70. Flores C, Degoutin S, Chai F, Raoul G, Hornez J-C, Martel B, et al. Gentamicin-loaded poly(lactic-co-glycolic acid) microparticles for the prevention of maxillofacial and orthopedic implant infections. Mater Sci Eng C Mater Biol Appl. 2016;(64):108–16.
71. Nichol T, Callaghan J, Townsend R, Stockley I, Hatton PV, Le Maitre C, et al. The antimicrobial activity and biocompatibility of a controlled gentamicin-releasing single-layer sol-gel coating on hydroxyapatite-coated titanium. Bone Joint J. 2021;103-B(3):522–9.
72. Cacaci M, Martini C, Guarino C, Torelli R, Bugli F, Sanguinetti M. Graphene oxide coatings as tools to prevent microbial biofilm formation on medical device. Adv Exp Med Biol. 2020;1282:21–35.
73. Dybowska-Sarapuk Ł, Kotela A, Krzemiński J, Wróblewska M, Marchel H, Romaniec M, et al. Graphene nanolayers as a new method for bacterial biofilm prevention: preliminary results. J AOAC Int. 2017;100(4):900–4.
74. Tahriri M, Del Monico M, Moghanian A, Tavakkoli Yaraki M, Torres R, Yadegari A, et al. Graphene and its derivatives: opportunities and challenges in dentistry. Mater Sci Eng C Mater Biol Appl. 2019;102:171–85.
75. Annunziata M, Oliva A, Basile MA, Giordano M, Mazzola N, Rizzo A, et al. The effects of titanium nitride-coating on the topographic and biological features of TPS implant surfaces. J Dent. 2011;39(11):720–8.
76. Scarano A, Piattelli M, Vrespa G, Caputi S, Piattelli A. Bacterial adhesion on titanium nitride-coated and uncoated implants: an in vivo human study. J Oral Implantol. 2003;29(2):80–5.
77. Wang J, An Y, Liang H, Tong Y, Guo T, Ma C. The effect of different titanium nitride coatings on the adhesion of Candida albicans to titanium. Arch Oral Biol. 2013;58(10):1293–301.
78. Kaluđerović MR, Schreckenbach JP, Graf H-L. Titanium dental implant surfaces obtained by anodic spark deposition—from the past to the future. Mater Sci Eng C Mater Biol Appl. 2016;69:1429–41.
79. Fröjd V, Linderbäck P, Wennerberg A, Chávez de Paz L, Svensäter G, Davies JR. Effect of nanoporous TiO_2 coating and anodized Ca2+ modification of titanium surfaces on early microbial biofilm formation. BMC Oral Health. 2011;11:8.
80. Benčina M, Resnik M, Starič P, Junkar I. Use of plasma technologies for antibacterial surface properties of metals. Molecules. 2021;26(5):1418.
81. Canullo L, Genova T, Wang H-L, Carossa S, Mussano F. Plasma of argon increases cell attachment and bacterial decontamination on different implant surfaces. Int J Oral Maxillofac Implants. 2017;32(6):1315–23.
82. Astaneh SH, Faverani LP, Sukotjo C, Takoudis CG. Atomic layer deposition on dental materials: processing conditions and surface functionalization to improve physical, chemical, and clinical properties—a Review. Acta Biomater. 2020;
83. Oral implant surfaces: Part 1—review focusing on topographic and chemical properties of different surfaces and in vivo responses to them—PubMed [Internet]. [cited 2020 Dec 20]. Available from: https://pubmed.ncbi.nlm.nih.gov/15543910/.

3D Printing—A Way Forward

6

Vinay Sivaswamy, Jukka P. Matinlinna, Vinicius Rosa, and Prasanna Neelakantan

Manufacture of any dental appliance, prostheses, or implants traditionally involves multiple fabrication methodologies, namely, but not limited to machining, casting, sanding, and finishing the products to their desired state. These processes are expensive, time-consuming and are heavily technique sensitive. Commercial production lines generally take a few weeks to months to produce dental implants because it involves turning a blank, machining it for threads, followed by surface treatment for optimising the surface design and completed with γ-irradiated sterilisation prior to packaging for mass distribution. A fully equipped dental laboratory with skilled technicians would require several days, sometimes weeks, to manufacture a dental implant prosthesis, be it metal or metal-free (zirconia, ZrO_2), to an optimal level for delivery to the dentist. The extended time is necessary for the technician to fabricate a pattern with minimal shrinkage and a smooth surface finish, which would allow for a copacetic casting with the passive fit. The manufactured framework is next sent to the clinician for verification of fit and is then sent back to the laboratory for ceramic layering and occlusal reconstruction, which is another time-consuming procedure. Each of these procedures needs to be stringently monitored due to the varying properties of the materials during manipulation, such as metal shrinkage, sag, and ceramic shrinkage.

Digital fabrication technologies allow us to completely bypass these limitations and enable the production of required objects in far less time but with superior levels of accuracy and precision. The design and production are completely computer controlled and are, thus, free of incidences of human errors. The only requirement is that clinicians and technicians need to be trained in the usage of these newer methods of fabrication [1].

Digital methods of fabrication can be grouped into two main categories, subtractive and additive. A subtractive method involves the use of CAD-CAM and CAM technology. CAD refers to 'computer-aided designing' and CAM refers to 'computer-aided machining' [1]. CAD-CAM is currently considered the gold standard technology for manufacturing dental prostheses in dental

V. Sivaswamy (✉)
Department of Prosthodontics and Implantology, Saveetha Dental College and Hospitals, Chennai, Tamil Nadu, India

J. P. Matinlinna
Dental Materials Science, Applied Oral Sciences and Community Dental Care, Faculty of Dentistry, The University of Hong Kong, Hong Kong SAR, People's Republic of China

Division of Dentistry, Faculty of Health Sciences, The University of Manchester, Manchester, UK

V. Rosa
Faculty of Dentistry, National University of Singapore, Singapore, Singapore

P. Neelakantan
Faculty of Dentistry, The University of Hong Kong, Hong Kong, Hong Kong

P. Neelakantan, A. Princy Solomon (eds.), *Dental Implants and Oral Microbiome Dysbiosis*,
https://doi.org/10.1007/978-3-030-99014-5_6

laboratories [2]. The prosthesis design is handled by either third-party software such as 3-Shape Dental Designer, ExoCAD, Blender for Dental or with proprietary software which come packaged with the milling unit such as CEREC from Dentsply Sirona [3, 5–7]. The milling units can be single purpose or highly versatile, depending on the number of axes the machining arms can traverse and the presence (or absence) of coolant spray. Zirconia and acrylic materials are usually dry milled without the use of coolant sprays. Dry milling units are also cost-effective and are the most common type of milling units employed by most dental laboratories. Wet milling, that is, the usage of coolant, is required for milling metals and glass ceramics and is more expensive compared to the dry milling units. These wet milling units also require more maintenance since the coolant residue needs to be routinely cleansed manually from the machine. Suction units are also required to be switched off during wet milling to prevent fluid aspiration into the suction unit and the risk of circuit shortage. Both dry milling and wet milling, however, produce prostheses with a high level of precision and at an exponentially faster rate compared to manual methods of manufacture. The current consensus is that CAD-CAM technology can be considered a superior method for manufacture of dental restorations or prosthesis [8].

Subtractive methods, however, are not without their limitations. CAD-CAM technology involves the milling of a blank or disc of the desired material in which the prostheses are to be fabricated. This involves a large amount of material wastage since the ground material cannot be reused again, especially in the case of zirconia and acrylic discs or blanks. The argument could be made that multiple prostheses can be milled out of a single disc. The fact remains, however, that there is still substantial material wastage that is unrecyclable. In the case of zirconia restorations, fully sintered or partially sintered discs may be reused. Fully sintered material is dense and subjects the milling tool to abrasion and confers microscopic cracks on the zirconia surface as well. These cracks could negatively affect the success rate of the restoration. Partially sintered material is easier to mill, however, it is subject to thermal changes during sintering, which could lead to discrepancies in adaptation [9]. Addressing these concerns is the counterpart to subtractive fabrication technology – additive fabrication, namely the technique known as 3D printing.

Today, 3D printing, at its core, refers to a compositional technique wherein an object is built up in successive layers. The layer thickness depends on the medium of the material used and the resolution rendered by the method of addition. An analogy to 3D printing would be the printing of images on a paper using an inkjet printer, which produces an image using controlled jetting of ink on the paper in two dimensions. That said, the same procedure is carried out by 3D printers, with the only difference being the application of the material in three dimensions as opposed to two. Design of the prostheses to be produced is carried out similarly to CAD-CAM technology with the use of dental designer software. Once the prosthesis is finalised, the digital file is transferred to a slicing software. Slicing software divides the digital object into multiple successive cross-sectional layers. As mentioned earlier, the thickness of these layers depends on the medium of the material used. The slices are typically 0.1 mm thick and are exported into a format that can be read by the 3D printer. Multiple file formats exist for 3D objects with the most common ones being STL, OBJ, and AMF formats [10]. The slicing software and file formats can be grouped into third-party solutions and proprietary software. Examples of third-party open-source slicing software include 3D Slicer, Cura from Ultimaker, Autodesk NetFabb and employ open-source file formats such as STL and OBJ [4, 11, 12]. Proprietary software are bundled with the 3D printer unit and use a different file format that can be read only by the company's own coupled 3D printer [13, 14]. In a bid to improve unification, most proprietary software, currently support the open-source file formats mentioned above.

3D printers were initially used to fabricate concept models. Concept models are non-functional and are simply a visual representation of a new design. Eventually, they were used to fabricate functional prototypes and are more sophisticated than a concept model. Functional prototypes usually take weeks to months to manufacture, which is dramatically cut short by the employment of 3D printers. The term 'rapid prototyping' hence came into play and is now synonymous with 3D printing fabrication. In the current timeline, 3D printing has been adopted by major global manufacturers to automate and hasten their production of commercial products. 3D printing has been adopted across various industries such as automobiles, aviation, clothing, jewellery, and dentistry.

6.1 History

Rapid prototyping, subsequently called 3D printing is considered an emerging technology that could eventually replace CAD-CAM methods as the gold standard for fabrication methodology. This technique, perhaps surprisingly, is not a new method and has been conceived and experimented on since the early 1980s (Fig. 6.1). The first documented proposal for 3D printing was in 1980 when Hideo Kodama applied for a patent on an XYZ plotter [15]. The patent was issued in 1981, however, a lack of interest in that niche resulted in a lack of research funds to further develop his technology and the endeavour was subsequently abandoned. The first patent considered as the foundation of the 3D printing industry belonged to Bill Masters in 1984. The stereolithography (STL) method of 3D printing also followed a similar pattern of introduction, wherein French inventors Alain Le Mehaute, Olivier De Witte, and Jean Claude Andre filed a patent for the process, which was later abandoned due to lack of interest. The method was once again developed and applied for by Charles Hull for which a patent was issued in 1986 and he popularised the technique by forming his own company, 3D Systems Corporation and marketed the first commercial 3D printer, the SLA-1. The STL file format was developed for the 3D systems' stereolithography printers, and it remains a popular choice for commercial usage even today.

The most common method of 3D printing is the fused deposition modelling (FDM), which was developed and patented by Scott Crump, who started his own company, Stratasys, in 1989, and which brought the first FDM machine to the commercial space in 1992. These two companies played a major role in further enhancement of 3D printing methodology through ongoing research and development [15, 16]. Yet, 3D printers remained a niche industrial fabrication method further restricted by the price, which commonly stretched above 100,000 USD. Major global manufacturers such as HP, Ricoh, Canon, and Toshiba have since then adopted and begun producing their own 3D printers, which have brought the cost down for mass commercial usage. 3D printers, nowadays, can be bought for less than 1000 USD, although the size and type of objects that can be produced are more basic and less functional in nature for these low-cost machines.

6.2 Techniques

There are currently several methods of 3D printing available with the most common method being the FDM technique mentioned above. The FDM technique, however, is not the most accurate technique, nor even the fastest method. That claim belongs to a variant of stereolithography, known as Nanojet printing. FDM and STL are the earliest techniques of 3D printing and are popular even today. There are several variants that have improved on those techniques and are entering the foray as their successors. The techniques used by each manufacturer for their variants of these archaic methods are labelled with newer, innovative terminologies which has resulted in multiple names for essentially the same methodology. An attempt has been made to classify 3D printing techniques by the International Organisation for Standardisation (ISO) and the American Society for Testing and Materials (ASTM) which is known as the ISO/ASTM 52900:2015 Additive Manufacturing standards (tabulated below in Table 6.1) [17, 18].

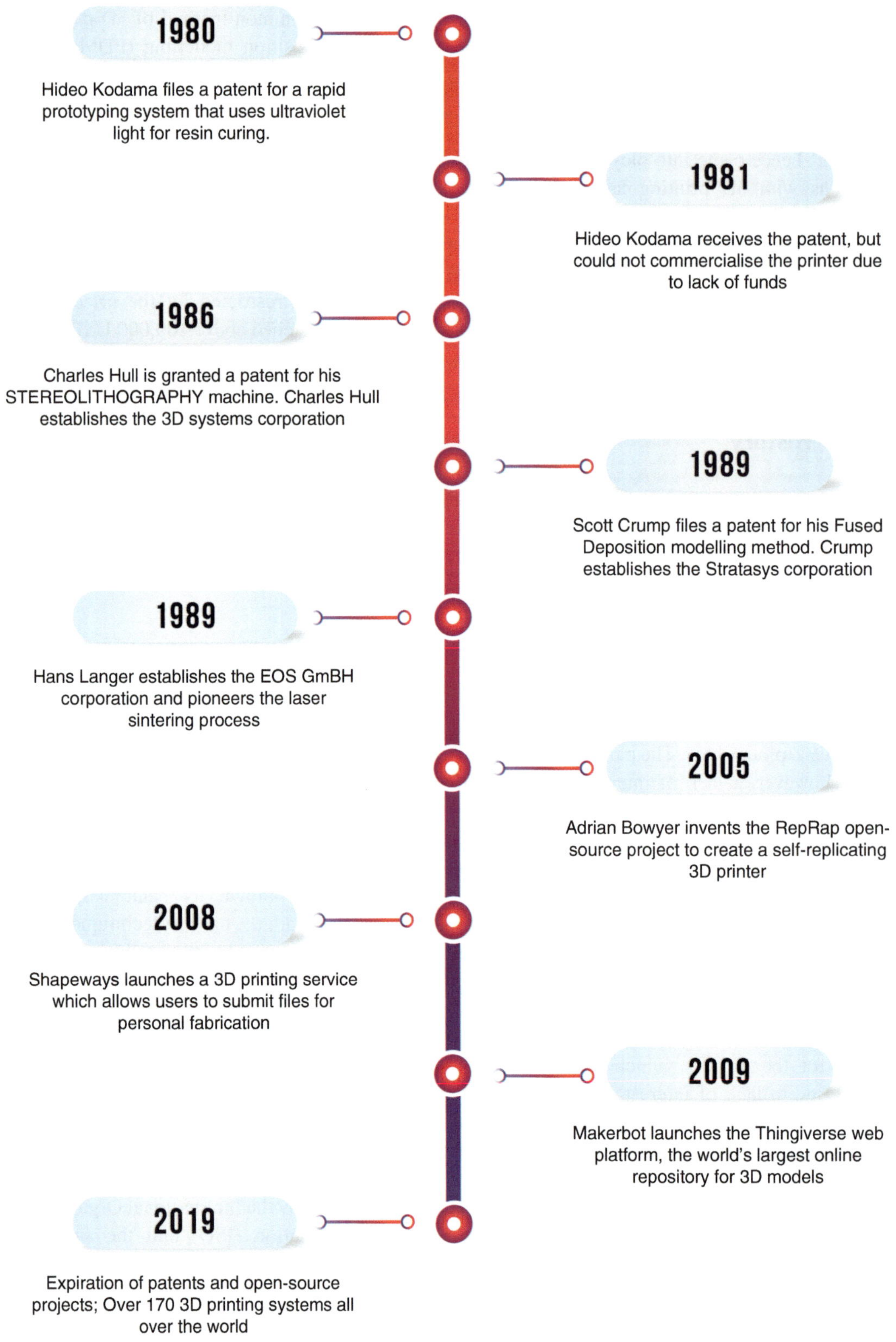

Fig. 6.1 Timeline of 3D printing

Table 6.1 Summary of 3D printing technology

3D printing technology	Description
Material extrusion	Extrusion of a molten material for build-up in successive layers
Vat photopolymerisation	Layer shape successively traced and solidified by a laser in a vat of liquid photopolymer
Material jetting	Deposition of liquid droplets that are cured by UV light/heat
Binder jetting	Successive layers of powder are fused by deposition of binder or adhesive
Powder bed fusion	Successive layers of powder are fused by a laser or a high energy heat source
Directed energy deposition	Successive layers of powder are fused by a layer as it is being deposited
Sheet lamination	Sheets of paper, plastic, or metal foil are fused together

Table 6.2 Categorisation of 3D printing technology

3D printing technology	Description
Material extrusion	Extrusion of a molten material for build-up in successive layers
Stereolithography	Layer shape successively traced and solidified by a laser in a vat of liquid photopolymer
Powder binding	Successive layers of powder are fused by a laser or a high energy heat source or a binder
Sheet lamination	Sheets of paper, plastic, or metal foil are fused together

The core method of 3D printing remains the same, that is, object fabrication based on the build-up of materials in thin, successive layers. The only difference between the various techniques is the medium of the material being used for fabrication. These methods (Table 6.2) can be grouped into four main categories based on their mechanism of action.

6.2.1 Anatomy of a 3D Printer

Before delving into the methodology, a description of the working parts of the 3D printer is necessary. Every 3D printer possesses two universal parts, namely the print head, and the build platform. The print head is a nozzle that delivers the material for fabrication. The print head may be coupled with a heating source or curing agent in some printers. The build platform is a base on which the material object is built. The platform may be submerged inside the material medium in some printers, namely the stereolithography models. Other components include a heat source or laser, movable mirrors that deflect lasers or light, which initiate curing, and an enclosure that surrounds the entire mechanism (Fig. 6.2). The enclosure may be orange tinted in stereolithography models to prevent unintentional premature curing of photosensitive resins [19].

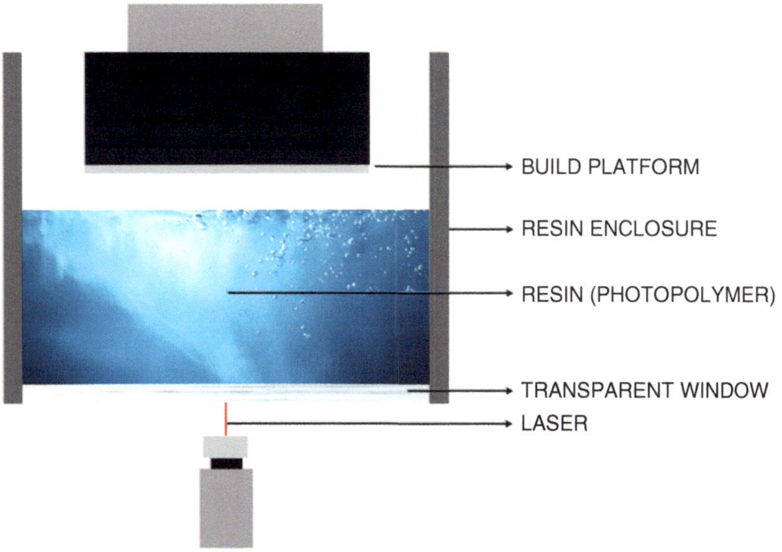

Fig. 6.2 Anatomy of a stereolithography based printer used in dentistry

6.3 Material Extrusion

Material extrusion has become the most common 3D printing methodology. It was invented by Scott Crump in 1989 and marketed by his company Stratasys in 1992 [15, 16]. This method employs thermoplastic filaments which are heated into a molten state as it is extruded through the print head nozzle. The molten material is laid down in a thin layer on the build platform as the print head moves in 2D space tracing and filling the shape of this layer. The material solidifies once laid on the build platform. The build platform is lowered down by the thickness of a single layer and the next layer of molten material is built on the previous layer (Fig. 6.3). This process is repeated till the entire object is completely built.

This method has been termed 'fused deposition modelling' by Stratasys and 'plastic jet printing' by 3D systems. Other terms for this method include 'fused filament modelling', 'melting and extruded modelling' and 'fused filament fabrication'. Earlier iterations of this method employed filaments of a single shade and were limited to an object of a single colour. There are multi-colour filaments available for material extrusion printers currently with more expensive machines such as the J850 from Stratasys, ProJet CJP series from 3D Systems, JetFusion 580 from HP, able to print professional full colour objects. Material extrusion produces objects with a layer thickness of approximately 0.1 mm, though less expensive machines produce thicker layers of 0.5 mm and above [20, 21].

6.3.1 Resins

Materials used for extrusion are commonly thermoplastic resins, such as acrylonitrile butadiene styrene (ABS), polyamides, acrylonitrile styrene acrylate, polyethylene terephthalate (PET), polycarbonate (PC), poly(methylmethacrylate) (PMMA), polyphenylsulfone (PPS), polyurethane (PU), polylactic acid (PLA), polycaprolactone (PCL), and polyhydroxyalkonate (PHA). PMMA, PC, PU, and PLA have been used in the production of healthcare devices in conjunction with gamma irradiation for sterilisation purposes [21]. Currently, there are resins with even antimicrobial properties such as AMultrax, and Copper 3D [22, 23]. Copper, silver, and zinc particles added to those resins have been observed to inhibit microbial growth.

6.3.2 Metals

Nickel-based alloys, titanium, and tantalum have been used for fabrication of metal objects through

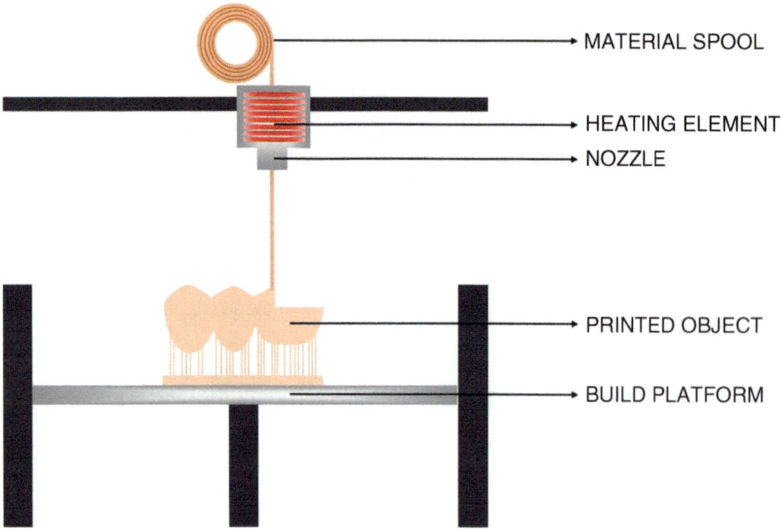

Fig. 6.3 Material extrusion method

material extrusion. A coil of thin metal wire is fed through the print head and heated to make it molten in order to build objects. There are two methods to make metal extrusion possible. One method is to use a metal alloy that possesses a low melting point. The other method is to use a different heating source to use commercial-scale metals such as titanium. The latter approach has employed arc fusion welding technology to heat titanium wire. This approach has been termed 'wire and arc additive manufacturing'. Another method to achieve the same is the usage of 'electron beam additive manufacturing' by Sciaky wherein an electron beam is used to fuse metal wires into the required parts. Rapid plasma deposition is another method to extrude a metal by melting, for example, a titanium wire in argon gas [24].

6.3.3 Composites

The materials described above are homogeneous with no additional constituent than the parent resin or metal. Various components have been added to the filament resin to improve their versatility and broaden their applications. Such composite materials have been listed below [25] (Table 6.3).

Table 6.3 Composite materials for extrusion-based printers

Constituents	Description
Resin + wood	Resin mixed with sawdust for the manufacture of wooden boards
Resin + brick	Produces objects with a sandstone finish
Resin + bronze	Resin mixed with bronze powder for products with a metallic finish
Resin + fibre	Resin mixed with carbon fibre for increased modulus of elasticity and bending resistance
Resin + carbon nanotubes	Resin reinforced with carbon nanotubes to impart electrostatic discharge protection
Resin + graphene	Resin mixed with graphene to improve electrical conductivity; graphene 3D labs showcased a 3D printed graphene battery
Resin + concrete	Resin mixed with cement, natural stone, and glass fibre to produce building material
Resin + clay	Resin mixed with liquid clay to produce ceramic
Resin + frosting	Resin mixed with flavoured frosting to produce edible printable confectionery

6.4 Vat Photopolymerisation

This method, vat polymerisation, employs a liquid photopolymer, which is cured by a light source, commonly a laser, to solidify successive layers of an object. Many variations of this method are employed by different manufacturers and are described below.

6.4.1 Stereolithography

Stereolithography was proposed by Charles Hull in 1986 and implemented in the SLA-1 3D printers marketed by his company, 3D Systems [15, 16]. A tank or vat of photosensitive polymer is solidified using a laser that traces the shape of each successive layer. There are two variations to the STL assembly. One model utilises a laser positioned over the vat of liquid polymer and the build platform below the vat but submerged inside. The build platform is lowered by the thickness of one single layer once the solidification of one layer is complete. A sweeping mechanism pushes a fresh layer of liquid polymer over the lower platform, which is cured by the laser and the entire process is repeated until fabrication is complete. The other model suspends the build platform over the polymer vat and is mechanically lowered to submerge the platform entirely inside the polymer during the commencement of fabrication. The laser is mounted below the vat, which is completely transparent to enable curing through the clear vat. The build platform, in this model, is raised by the thickness of one layer once the solidification of a layer is complete. This method can be termed 'inverted stereolithography' (Fig. 6.4). On completion, the fabricated object needs to be removed from the build platform and cleansed of the liquid residues. This cleansing is performed using a solvent such as 90% isopropyl alcohol,

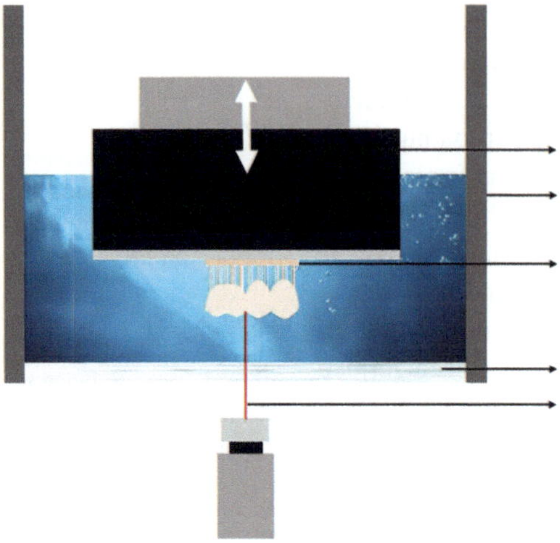

Fig. 6.4 Mechanism of a stereolithography printer used in dentistry

followed by rinsing with water. Certain objects may require further curing using an UV curing chamber. Stereolithography is typically more precise and produces objects with thinner layers at approximately 25–50 μm. It has to be kept in mind that the liquid polymer material costs more than the thermoplastic filaments required for material extrusion. The liquid polymer falls within a price range of 150 to 400 USD for lower-end machines whereas thermoplastic filaments range between 40 and 50 USD and upwards [26].

6.4.1.1 Continuous Liquid Interface Production

This method is similar to inverted stereolithography, albeit a layer of uncured resin is positioned between the bottom of the vat and the solidified layer with a dead zone that is exposed to oxygen. This uncured resin layer is maintained below the object as each layer is cured maintaining the so-called continuous liquid interface. This method has been developed and employed by Carbon 3D [27].

6.4.2 Digital Light Processing

Digital light processing (DLP) is a variant of vat photopolymerisation in which an imaging chip containing an array of miniature movable mirrors is used to reflect light from a projector on to the photopolymer for solidification. In other words, a projector and mirrors reflect light for curing instead of a laser. The other difference is that the entire layer is cured in a single instance instead of tracing the outline and filling in the layer. The projector lens projects an image of the entire layer, which is reflected by the mirrors on the photopolymer. The entire layer is solidified en masse and is therefore theoretically faster than the STL method. There are a few variants of the DLP method, one of which is the moving light system that employs a projector mounted over the vat of photopolymer and needs UV light for faster curing of the polymer. Another variant is the daylight polymer printing (DPP) method that utilises LCD panels to project entire object layers and also uses natural light instead of UV light for curing [28](Table 6.4).

Table 6.4 Digital light processing technology

DLP variants	Mechanism of action
Moving light	Projector is mounted over the polymer vat and employs UV light for faster curing
Daylight polymer printing	Utilises LCD panels to project entire object layers and employs natural light for curing
Scan, spin, and selective photocure	Reflects light off a spinning drum and is then passed through optical elements on to the polymer
Lithography based ceramic manufacturing	DLP method on a photopolymer containing ceramic particles

6.4.3 Two-Photon Polymerisation

This advanced method allows for the production of objects on the nanoscale. The two-photon polymerisation (2PP) method utilises a femtosecond (fs) pulsed laser to emit photons on a specialised photopolymer containing highly specific initiators and solidifies only on contact with two photons simultaneously. Since this is possible only at the centre portion of the laser beam, it allows for precise fabrication throughout the polymer vat rather than simply the surface layer. The resolution achieved with this method is from 200 nm to 400 nm in the XY axes and is exponentially faster with manufacture speeds at 100 mm/s. A commercial 3D printer using the 2PP method is available from a German manufacturer Nanoscribe, the Photonic Professional GT2. The applications with this model extend to the biomedical area in addition to electrical system parts. The only caveat is that this method currently cannot produce objects larger than 100 mm [29–31].

6.5 Material Jetting

This method is similar to inkjet style printing in which the polymer is sprayed from the print head nozzle and is subsequently cured using UV light (Fig. 6.5). This method has been termed 'PolyJet' from Stratasys and 'MultiJet Printing' from 3D systems [32, 33]. The variants of material jetting are listed below (Table 6.5).

6.6 Powder Binding

This method refers to the fabrication of an object using powdered material, which is successively layered. There are three variants under this category.

6.6.1 Binder Jetting

This method is also termed 'inkjet powder printing' or 'Z printing' since it relates to laying down material along the Z axis. The technology was

Table 6.5 Material jetting technology

Material jetting variants	Description
Wax deposition modelling	Wax material is sprayed from the print head nozzle for the fabrication of wax patterns
Printoptical	The polymer droplets can be individually per droplet or left uncured for smoothness
Nanoparticle jetting	Liquid suspension containing metal particles is sprayed and heat is used to sinter the metal particles together in the desired shape

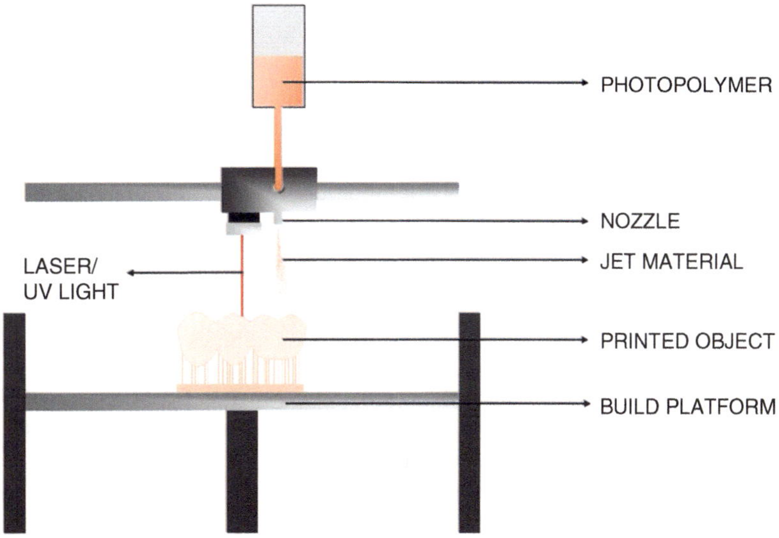

Fig. 6.5 Material jetting method

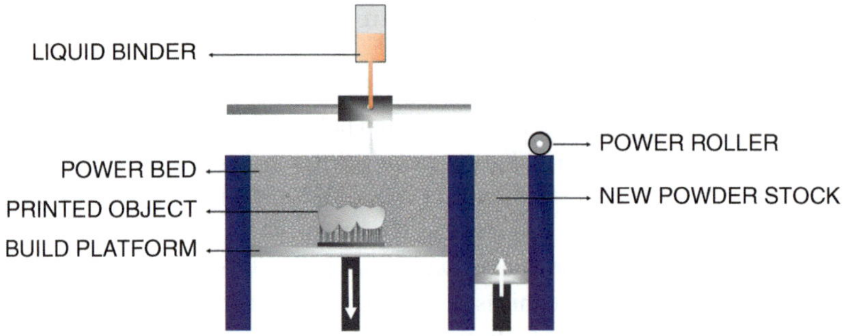

Fig. 6.6 Binder jetting method

developed by the Massachusetts Institute of Technology (MIT) and was adopted by Z-Corporation and ExOne. The powdered material is stored in a mechanised platform that can be termed the powder reservoir. The reservoir is slightly elevated, and a sweeping mechanism (or a roller) sifts a thin layer of powder into the print bed. A print head nozzle then sprays the binder material in the shape of the first layer. Once the binder solidifies it fuses the material in the first layer. The platform is again elevated, and the roller sifts the next layer of powder on top of the first layer followed by spraying the binder. This process is repeated until the entire object is completely fabricated (Fig. 6.6). Following completion, the object remains surrounded by loose powder which requires removal. Most printers are equipped with a de-powdering chamber that employs high-powered vacuum systems to remove the excess powder surrounding the object [32, 34, 35).

6.6.1.1 Gypsum

Binder jetting employs gypsum-based powder and the binder is usually water, which sets the material into a plaster object. Gypsum products are very porous, friable, and brittle upon completion. This is referred to as the 'green state'. Upon completion of the object, post processing methods such as infiltration and baking are required to improve the strength of the product. The object is infiltrated with wax or resin to seal the porous gypsum substructure and is subsequently baked, if required. The binder can be mixed with dyes in order to impart colour to the object. Binder jetting is commonly used to produce concept models or casting moulds. Moulds are produced by using an investment material (casting sand), a refractory variant of gypsum plaster [36, 37].

6.6.1.2 Metals

Metal products can also be fabricated using the binder jetting method. Powders containing a mix of iron, bronze, chrome, and aluminium are available. The binder material is sprayed onto a layer of the metal powder and binds the metal particles together. A heating system dries the bound layer, and the next layer of powder is laid down. Once the fabrication is complete, the object is transferred to a curing oven which hardens the binder further. Infiltration of the porous object is carried out net where the object is placed in a kiln containing aluminium oxide grit and heated to over 2000 °C to liquefy the metal powder and fill the porous object. On cooling, the object is sanded and polished to a smooth surface [32, 35].

6.6.1.3 Ceramics

The same technology can also be used to fabricate ceramic objects by replacing the metal powder with alumina (Al_2O_3) and silica (SiO_2). The ceramic powder is bounded layer-wise using the binding agent. The object is cured to evaporate moisture and harden the binder. The object is then sintered in a furnace to harden it [36].

6.6.1.4 Glass Printing

Glass objects can also be produced using the binder jetting technology, following the same methodology as mentioned previously. Powdered soda lime glass is used in layers and adhered using a binder. The object is cured in an oven and de-powdered. This is followed by infiltrating the object with more glass by firing it in a kiln containing glass powder.

6.6.2 Powder Bed Fusion

Metal objects produced using binder jetting are porous and may not achieve homogeneity or complete solidification even after infiltration and sintering. Complete solidification is possible when the metal powder particles are fused together rather than bound using an adhesive. This procedure is known as laser sintering. The methodology is similar to binder jetting wherein the metal powder is swept from a reservoir using a sweeping mechanism onto the print bed. Instead of a binding adhesive, a laser traces the shape of the first layer on the metal powder. The high-intensity laser beam heats the metal powder and enables the fusion of each granule together. The next layer of powder is swept onto the solidified layer and the process is repeated (Fig. 6.7). De-powdering is required to remove the excess unfused powder from the completed object. Laser sintering can be used to produce objects in wax, resins, ceramics, and metals. The metal powders used for this procedure are finely ground and are approximately 20 µm in size. The powder should be spherical to enable flowability and is usually manufactured using inert gas atomisation.

Two component materials are also available with differing melting points that allow faster completion of the sintering process for each layer. One example is 'alumide', nylon powder mixed with aluminium which produces objects with a metallic finish. High accuracy with a resolution of approximately 80 µm is achievable with this method. This method is also termed direct metal laser sintering (DMLS), selective laser sintering (SLS), and direct metal printing (DMP). A neodymium yttrium aluminium garnet (Nd:YAG) laser is employed in this method to selectively melt the metal powder into a thin layer. The temperature achieved by the laser to melt the powder, however, does not reach the melting point of the metal used and simply sinters the metal powder together instead of complete melting [38, 39].

6.6.2.1 Selective Laser Melting (SLM)

This method is a variant of the SLS technique and it employs a CO_2 or Nd:YAG laser to fully melt the metal powder in an inert gas atmosphere (argon or nitrogen). The thermal changes in this method result in internal stresses in the completed object. These stresses are relieved by heat treatment post-production [38, 40–42].

6.6.2.2 Electron Beam Melting (EBM)

A variant of powder bed fusion, this method, electron beam melting (EBM), employs an electron beam to fuse metal granules, instead of a laser beam. The chamber is preheated to 700 °C to minimize thermal changes in the object. A tungsten filament is heated to 3000 °C for the production of electrons. The electrons are focussed into a beam using magnetic coils. The electron beam passes over the layer in the print bed multiple times. The electron first preheats the build material at the first pass followed by melting the outline of the layer with the second pass. More passes are made to completely melt the

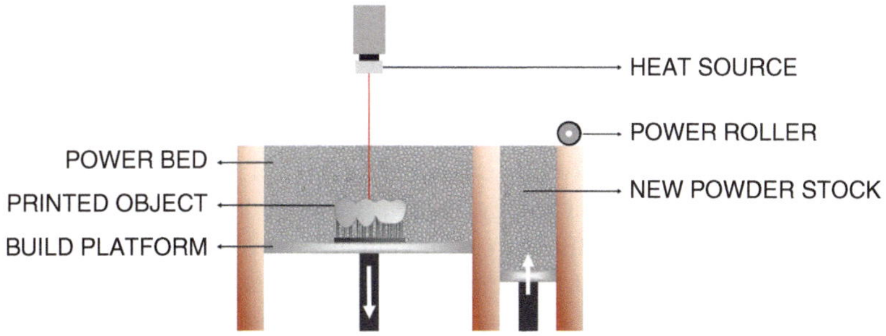

Fig. 6.7 Powder bed fusion method

metal powder inside the outline. The entire procedure is performed in a vacuum environment with purified argon to prevent contamination. The electron beam is moved around using electromagnetic deflection. The method is currently used for high-value materials such as titanium and cobalt-chrome [43–45].

6.6.2.3 Selective Heat Sintering (SHS)

A thermal print head is used to simultaneously lay down and solidify plastic powder in layers. SHS produces objects in 100 μm thickness and is an alternative to material extrusion since it requires far fewer components. It is also cost-effective since it does not require a laser [46].

6.6.3 Directed Energy Deposition

This method is also known as laser powder forming, laser metal deposition, and laser engineered net shaping. A motion-controlled print head directs metal powder into a high-power laser beam to melt it and is layered on a build platform that is also motion controlled. Since both print head and build platform are movable, the fabrication doesn't need to be made in successive layers and can even be applied to a layer material on prefabricated objects for modification or repair purposes [47].

6.7 Sheet Lamination

Laminated object manufacture (LOM) advances a sheet of build material to the build platform and adheres it to a substrate using a heated roller. A laser or blade cuts the outline of the object layer in the sheet. The excess material outside the outline is cross-hatched to facilitate easy removal following completion. The next sheet is layered on the previous layer and the same process is repeated. This method was invented by Helisys in 1991 and is currently implemented in printers from MCor technology, which have modified lamination machines to use commonly available A4 copier paper for object fabrication [48, 49].

6.7.1 Ultrasonic Additive Manufacturing

A variant of LOM which employs high-frequency vibrations at 20,000 Hz to fuse layers of a metal tape into a block that is cut into shape using a laser [50, 51].

6.8 Stepping

The layered method of fabrication produces objects which have identifiable 'steps' across their surface on completion. The elimination of these visible steps can be achieved by either using a printer with a resolution of less than 10 μm or by employing some post-processing sanding or milling. Metals and resin objects require milling post-production in order to cut away the support structures and impart a smooth surface texture.

6.9 Support Structures

Products made with 3D printing are subject to a technical complication during the manufacturing process wherein overhanging parts require additional support to be held in place during the layering. Support platforms or 'rafts' are generated by the slicer software prior to additive manufacturing. The rafts' dimensions can be adjusted by the operator according to their preference. The raft junctions are usually set at 0.5 mm to ease separation from the manufactured object. Rafts can usually be broken manually from the object or precisely incised using a sharp plier. This method of support is known as 'breakaway support technology' (BST). There are also printers that use a secondary print head to print support structures in soluble material such as polyvinyl acetate (PVA). These soluble structures can be separated from the object by dissolution in a tank of water. This method is known as 'soluble support technology' (SST). Support platforms can be avoided when binder jetting and powder bed fusion methods are used for the production of non-metallic objects since the tank of uncured powder secures the solidified object in place till all layers are complete [52].

6.10 Post-Processing

3D printed objects usually require post-production finishing procedures due to stepping and a rough surface resulting from the separation of the supporting rafts. Liquid-based methods such as stereolithography require cleansing the object of residual material using isopropyl alcohol. Resin-based objects are also subject to curing for complete photopolymerisation followed by finishing procedures. The finishing procedures commonly employed are sandblasting, manual abrasion, electropolishing, computer numeric control (CNC) milling, and laser polishing based on the material used for fabrication [53, 54].

6.11 Application in Implant Dentistry

The layer-wise control and precision presented by additive manufacturing (AM) lend itself naturally to the manufacture of dental prostheses, especially dental subgingival implant restorations. Dental restorations require calibration and finesse in the μm range since the tactile threshold for occlusal contacts extends till 20 μm. Any restoration that possesses premature contacts above 20 μm will be perceptible to individuals and has the potential to cause occlusal disharmony and physical distress. This perception applies itself doubly so for implant retained restorations due to the lack of shock-absorbing periodontal ligaments around the implants [55, 56]. Digital workflow promises precision manufacturing which could improve accuracy of the final restorations as well as reduced manufacturing duration. Additive manufacturing (AM) also extends to manufacture of the implant body and not just the restorative component. AM applications in dental manufacturing are listed in the table below (Table 6.6).

Table 6.6 Applications of 3D printing in implant dentistry

Category	Applications
Treatment planning	Guided placement stents Mock models for practice and visualisation
Treatment	Provisional crowns and bridges Definitive crowns and bridges Implant fixture Implant frameworks Dentures
Education	Models for visualisation

6.11.1 Guided Placement Stents

Stents for implant placement were initially hard splints with holes to aid in marking osteotomy sites prior to implant placements. These stents did not account for anatomy and contour of the residual ridge and were extremely limited during stage I implant surgery. Guiding stents are currently manufactured using a combination of cone-beam computed tomography (CBCT), implant planning software, and additive manufacturing technology. CBCT aids in three-dimensional acquisition of volumetric data of the residual ridge in the digital imaging and communications in medicine (DICOM) format. The DICOM files aid in 3D reconstruction of the entire maxilla and mandible. Implant planning software (Implant Planning Studio, 3Shape; SIMPLANT Studio, Materialise Medical) allows the import of these DICOM files and enables the visualisation of implants in the desired regions. The exact dimensions and shapes of implants are made available as digital files by each manufacturer for use in planning software. Clinicians or laboratory technicians requiring a specific implant system would need to download the appropriate digital files of that system to the library (database) of their planning software. Measurements of the ridge in the region of the missing tooth are estimated and the chosen implant is virtually positioned in the most optimal configuration. The software generates the stent around the virtually positioned implant. These stents are generated with openings to attach manufacturer-specific metal sleeves to aid in drill positioning during osteotomy. These stents can be customised to either allow multiple drills throughout the osteotomy procedure or to guide only the pilot drill to initiate the stage 1 procedure.

Guided surgical kits that allow different sizes of metal sleeves to be attached to the surgical guide are available from each manufacturer. Vertical stoppers are also available to control osteotomy in the vertical plane. It has been established from literature that surgical guides are able to minimise deviations in the horizontal plane. Deviations in the vertical plane as well as in the palatal aspect (for upper anterior implants) are still possible and need to be actively monitored during implant placement. Guided placements are currently considered the gold standard method of stage 1 implant surgery. A few limitations to this method are the added cost for manufacturing the stent and the extended duration required for stent fabrication. Placement stents are usually fabricated using the stereolithography method [57–59].

6.11.2 Models

Dental models or casts can be fabricated for the purpose of visualisation as well as manual practice prior to implant placement. These models can serve to educate patients as well as dental students. Models can be made with the soft tissue layer intact or can be made at the bone level using DICOM file integration for 3D reconstruction of the maxilla or mandible. Implant analogues or mock implants can be drilled and positioned into these models to determine the optimal drill position for implant placement in order to prevent the incidence of bone fenestration. It has been established in literature that implant positioning is improved when clinicians undertake prior practice in osteotomy using printed bone level models [60–63].

6.11.3 Crowns and Bridges

Bridge and crowns can be printed in a wide variety of materials using additive manufacturing techniques. Provisional restorations can be made using PMMA resin and definitive restorations can be made using cobalt-chrome alloys or alumina particles. Stereolithography method is used for resin material and selective laser sintering is used for metal restorations. 3D printed ceramic restorations have not yet reached routine commercial usage in clinical practice due to the cost of the material. There are in vitro studies in which ceramic restorations have already been fabricated and tested using additive manufacturing methods such as material extrusion, binder jetting, as well as stereolithography methods. In vitro evaluations have found such restorations to be clinically acceptable when compared with conventionally manufactured restorations [64–66]. Processing a ceramic material using AM methods requires the monitoring of certain parameters, which have been summarised by Methani et al. [67]. The parameters used for processing ceramics have been listed in the table below (Table 6.7). These crowns and bridges, as well as titanium implants, can be surface treated with subtractive methods such as etching and grit-blasting or subjected to additive methods such as a silane coating to further improve their adhesive bond with the underlying substructure [68–70].

As shown in Table 6.7, the parameters differ for each method due to the state of the material used (liquid or solid) and the method used for solidification for powder-based methods.

Production of ceramic objects using AM techniques relies on a resin material mixed with ceramic particles. Stereolithographic techniques are dependent on the particle size, slurry viscosity, and dry matter content in the slurry. The dry matter content should be more than 50% by volume in order to withstand thermal changes during sintering without cracking. The dry matter content can be increased by utilising particle sizes from 0.5 μm to 2 μm, with 1.5 μm alumina particles producing acceptable clinical crowns in a study by Dehurtevent et al. [71]. Moreover, Marion et al. have observed that stereolithography manufactured alumina crowns with high dry matter content and large particle sizes possess high Weibull modulus indicating structural reliability and flexural strength. Marginal adaptation

Table 6.7 Processing parameters for 3D printing ceramics

Category	Parameters	Values
Stereolithography	Particle size	0.5–1.5 μm
	Slurry viscosity	Low Zeta potential
	Dry matter	70–80%
Material extrusion	Critical nozzle height	840 μm
	pH	7.0–7.5
	Slurry viscosity	High Zeta potential
Powder bed fusion	Laser power	21 W
	Scan speed	1800 mm/s
	Scan spacing	0.1 mm/s
Material jetting	Ohnesorge number for liquid	0.1–1
	Printhead distance	Close to platform
Binder jetting	Power level	60%
	Binder saturation level	50%

was also found to be equal to those of milled restorations indicating that stereolithography manufactured crowns can be used in routine clinical cases.

Material extrusion methods rely on a paste like slurry which is dependent on the Zeta potential, a function of the material pH. A higher Zeta potential indicates high stability and the ability to resist aggregation. Slurries with pH of 7.0–7.5 have been found to possess pseudoplastic behaviour and demonstrated reduced viscosity with increasing shear rates, in a study conducted by Wang et al. Another crucial parameter is the critical nozzle height, a level of balance between the nozzle height (the distance between build platform and print head nozzle) and nozzle speed, diameter, and extrusion rate. Wang et al. have found 840 μm as the ideal critical nozzle height for a nozzle speed of 4.25 mm/s, diameter of 0.7 mm, and extrusion at the rate of 2.5 10^{-3} cm^3/s [72].

Powder bed fusion methods rely on sintering powder particles using a laser. Agglomeration of the powder particles is enhanced by increasing the binder content. Laser power should be sufficient to generate an energy density high enough to fuse the metal particles. Laser power is inversely associated with the scan speed and scan spacing. Low scan speeds increase the exposure of the particle to the laser beam resulting in higher agglomeration. Scan spacing refers to the duration between consecutive passes of the beam. Reducing the scan spacing has the same effect as reduced scan speeds.

Material jetting relies on layer wise deposition of material dispersed as droplets from the print head nozzle. Material jetting depends on the Ohnesorge (Oh) number, which refers to the viscosity of the dispersed material. An Oh number between 0.1 and 1 is considered ideal for jetting. Binder jetting relies on the deposition of the binder or adhesive to bind the powder substrate. The major parameters for binder jetting are power and saturation level. Power refers to the intensity of heat applied to cure the binder and saturation refers to the content of binder dispersed through the print head [73].

6.11.4 Implant Frameworks

A plethora of novel restorative solutions are made possible due to the advent of implant dentistry. Implants can be used to replace a single missing tooth or the entire dentition and associated structures. Crowns and bridges for dental implants are fabricated in a similar manner to those of tooth-supported prostheses. Full mouth prostheses, however, are more tedious to fabricate and require a high level of technical mastery from both the clinician and the laboratory personnel. Such extensive restorations are also highly time-consuming and are expensive to produce. Additive manufacturing methods have the potential to eliminate all such problems and are capable of producing frameworks with a high degree of passivity and accurate marginal fit. The earliest iteration of incorporating digital workflow into the fabrication of implant frameworks involved a combination of additive manufacture and lost wax casting methods. A resin pattern of the implant framework was fabricated, which was converted to metal using the lost wax casting procedure. This approach did reduce the chance of pattern deformation and shrinkage incident with manual fabrication but did not reduce the incidence of distortion associated with thermal changes during casting. Currently, implant frameworks can be produced en masse using additive manufacture without having to resort to a combined approach. Powder bed fusion methods have been successfully used to produce entire metal frameworks with a high degree of precision [74–77]. Zirconia frameworks for full mouth rehabilitation, however, have not yet been produced using additive manufacture and are still in the experimental stage. CAD-CAM methods are still the gold standard for manufacturing zirconia frameworks. SLS, SLM, and EBM methods have been used to manufacture frameworks of titanium or cobalt-chrome alloy. Customised titanium meshes for guided bone regeneration have also been produced and successfully used to treat patients with bone defects. Scientific evidence on the use of customised titanium meshes for treatment of bone defects by Inoue et al. and Sumida et al. support the implementation of this method as a standard treatment protocol for regenerative cases [78, 79].

6.11.5 Dental Implant Fixtures

Implant fixtures can be fabricated following the conventional threaded design or as a root form analogue replicating the shape of the missing root. Successful instances of using SLS and SLM implants have been documented with high success rates and enhanced bone growth around these implants. A retrospective study by Cerea and Dolcini revealed a 98% success rate in 70 patients treated with AM titanium implants 2 years following restoration. Subperiosteal implant fixtures made with AM techniques have also been used as a successful treatment modality as reported by Mangano et al. Moreover, Che et al. have reported the use of customised large diameter implants for the treatment of bony defects in an animal model study. The AM implants have demonstrated high bone ingrowth, increased trabecular thickness, and high bone mineral density due to the porous surface of these implants. Osteoblasts have been observed to adhere to nanostructured scaffolds and pits far more effectively than to microstructures. The nanogeometry produced as a result of AM methods, therefore, renders the implant surface osseoinductive. Histomorphometric studies have shown that SLM implants with a pore size of 350 μm demonstrate high levels of cell growth, migration, and adhesion (stabilisation). Another benefit of the AM implant is the reduced modulus of elasticity of these fixtures. Stress shielding is a mechanical problem associated with conventional titanium implants due to the high elastic modulus of the fixture. Cortical and cancellous bone have lower elastic moduli when compared with titanium and this discrepancy results in irregular and uneven force distribution to the surrounding bone. The AM titanium implants possess a highly interconnected porous structure that reduces the elastic modulus drastically, with the value closer to that of natural bone and improving the functionality and force distribution patterns of these implants [80, 81]. Furthermore, these custom-manufactured implants may be designed to inhibit biofilm formation by tethering silanes and other polymers to their surface [82–85].

6.11.6 Dentures

Dentures are a common and affordable mode of replacing missing dentition. The combination of dentures with implant therapy has rendered the modality highly versatile and cost-effective for patients who cannot afford more expensive fixed therapy. Dentures can be made removable with the use of attachments on implants or can be fully attached to a substructure and secured firmly to implants (hybrid dentures). Denture processing methods namely compression moulding and injection moulding are technique sensitive and highly time-consuming. Stereolithography and DLP methods have been used to fabricate complete dentures. Using additive manufacturing eliminates the need for manual teeth arrangement and reduces the production time. AM dentures have shown clinically acceptable levels of fit and are currently available for commercial usage in clinical practice. In vitro studies have shown high levels of precision and trueness of 3D-printed dentures. Such dentures can be made as a monoblock prosthesis with both denture teeth and base produced as a single unit or as two components with separate denture teeth and the denture base. The monoblock denture is imparted gingival colour and characterisation using indirect resin composites. The two-component system can be produced using pink colour resin for the denture base and tooth coloured resin for the denture teeth. The denture base is produced with recesses for attaching denture teeth. Flowable bonding resins are available for attaching denture teeth to the denture base. Denture fabrication is rapidly gaining ground as more commercial manufacturers have begun to promote the method as a faster and convenient method bypassing the time requirement for manual fabrication [86–90].

6.12 Future Trends

6.12.1 Bioprinting

The methods discussed so far describe the fabrication of inorganic objects. The true potential of 3D printing, however, lies in its versatility, with the foray of additive manufacture into the realm of synthetic biology heralding a new era in healthcare technology. 3D printers capable of fabricating organic tissue by controlling the placement of layers of living cells have been developed by a few manufacturers across the world [91].

Makoto Nakamura, a Japanese paediatrician, developed the first printer capable of jetting living cells encased in sodium alginate hydrogel into a calcium chloride solution. Nakamura had experimented with a standard photo printer earlier where he faced the issue of cells clogging up the printer. His collaboration with Epson resulted in the first printer capable of outputting living cells. Further research led to the creation of a bio-printer that could create biotubes, a replacement material for blood vessels [92, 93].

Moreover, Gabor Forgacs had developed a printer capable of building tissue from clumps of bio-ink spheroids which contained thousands of cells. Forgacs founded Organovo in 2007 to create tissue on demand for research and surgical applications. Their collaboration with Invetech resulted in the Novogen MMX, a commercial bioprinter, containing multiple print heads which are loaded with bio-ink spheroids. The second print head outputs a bio paper support for producing a scaffold to support the dispersed cells. A biopsy from the patient is required to source a sample of cells. These are cultured in growth medium to increase the volume of cells for the production of the bio-ink spheroid. Production of the spheroid is dependent on the tissue to be built. If the tissue to be printed is a blood vessel, a cluster of endothelial cells and fibroblasts are compressed into a tubed shaped specimen that is sliced into small pieces forming the bio-ink spheroids. These spheroids are loaded into the print head and the second print head lays down bio-paper, a structure made from water, collagen, and gelatine [94].

Organovo supplies synthetic tissue to pharmaceutical companies to test their new drugs without the use of animal experiments or routine in vitro models which are not representative of the in vivo condition. Currently, human liver and kidney tissues are manufactured using the process described above. Research is ongoing on the production of synthetic skin, thyroid tissue, and entire organs [95].

EnvisionTEC, a company popular in the dental fraternity, for their DLP printers, has produced the 3D-Bioplotter, a printer capable of building custom scaffolds using bio-ink spheroids as well as biodegradable polymers such as polycaprolactone and polylactic acid. These scaffolds could be used for guided bone regeneration for the treatment of bone defects. Xillogic (The Netherlands) and Next 21 (Japan) are working on a calcium phosphate bone analogue, termed CT bone, which could be used to replace damaged bone. The CT bone aims to avoid graft rejection issues and could be a replacement for particulate grafts in dentistry. These products are still in the experimental stage and require further testing for extrapolation to commercial clinical usage [96].

6.12.1.1 In Vivo Bioprinting

Nevertheless, research is underway on the application of bioprinting in the direct repair of wounds. The process utilises fibroblasts and keratinocytes to spray on the wound and form a new layer of skin [97]. Another development in the realm of in vivo bioprinting comes from Australian researchers from the ARC Centre of Excellence for Electromaterials Science (ACES), in the form of a 'Bio-Pen'. This device aims to allow surgeons to layer cells on damaged areas directly to accelerate their regeneration. The biopen dispenses cells suspended in polymer hydrogels. The polymer is solidified with UV light as the cells are laid down to act as a scaffold [98]. Both methods of bioprinting are currently being investigated on their applicability in real-life situations.

As research progresses in these fields, it may be possible to insert custom fabricated titanium implants as a root form analogue in the region of the missing tooth and use bioprinting to lay down inorganic calcium phosphate to accelerate bone formation around the implant. Another feasibility would be the dispersal of calcium phosphate material into the alveolar socket in the shape of the root and crown to form a fully synthetic tooth in vivo [99].

6.12.2 Nanotechnology

Manufacture of objects within a scale of 1–100 nm can be considered nanotechnology. The premise of using nanotechnology is to manipulate and control individual atoms and molecules to custom fabricate functional structures. Functionally graded structures that have unique properties similar to biologic tissue is made possible through the application of nanotechnology. Biologic tissues are not homogenous and consist of different phases and constituents, which serve different functions under a multitude of conditions. Cortical and cancellous bones are a prime example of natural functional grading. Producing the same gradient in synthetic objects such as implants (and their coatings) would render the implants strong enough to withstand occlusal loads as well as prevent stress shielding along with an improvement in biocompatibility [100–102]. There have been studies investigating different combinations of materials for dental implants, namely titanium with hydroxyapatite (HAp), titanium nitride (TiN) and zirconia [103, 104]. These combinations have proven effective in in vitro conditions and are under testing for clinical usage. Current application of nanotechnology is the fabrication of carbon nanotubes, which are used to reinforce glass or plastics to increase material strength. These nanocomposites are a combination of ABS, PLA, and TPU with graphene to produce a single atom thick lattice. The methods that are capable of printing in the nanometre scale are Nanojet printing and Two photon polymerisation. These methods are restricted to experimental niche production currently due to the sophisticated equipment required as well as the expense of manufacture. One must keep in mind that the 'conventional' 3D printers that are currently available at less than 1000 USD were in the hundred-thousand-dollars range during their first iteration. The current 3D printing processes will bring down manufacturing costs even further, which will make the production of sophisticated equipment for advanced processes, including bioprinting and nano-printing, more cost-effective.

Conflict of InterestThe authors are not affiliated to any of the commercial manufacturers or firms mentioned in this chapter or are sponsored, in any thinkable way, for the active promotion or marketing of any product related to 3D printing.

References

1. Dawood A, Marti Marti B, Sauret-Jackson V, Darwood A. 3D printing in dentistry. Br Dent J. 2015;219(11):521–9.
2. Papadiochou S, Pissiotis AL. Marginal adaptation and CAD-CAM technology: a systematic review of restorative material and fabrication techniques. J Prosthet Dent. 2018;119(4):545–51.
3. 3Shape software—Dental CAD/CAM solutions for labs and clinics [Internet]. 3Shape. [cited 2021 Oct

5]. Available from: https://www.3shape.com/en/software-overview
4. 3D Slicer image computing platform [Internet]. 3D Slicer. [cited 2021 Oct 5]. Available from: https://slicer.org/.
5. Carina. exocad DentalCAD—exocad [Internet]. [cited 2021 Oct 5]. Available from: https://exocad.com/our-products/exocad-dentalcad.
6. Digital Dentistry Software [Internet]. Blenderfordental. [cited 2021 Oct 5]. Available from: https://www.blenderfordental.com
7. Design with CEREC | Dentsply Sirona [Internet]. [cited 2021 Oct 5]. Available from: https://www.dentsplysirona.com/en-nz/categories/cerec/design-with-cerec.html.
8. Alghazzawi TF. Advancements in CAD/CAM technology: options for practical implementation. J Prosthodont Res. 2016;60(2):72–84.
9. No-Cortes J, Ayres AP, Lima JF, Markarian RA, Attard NJ, Cortes ARG. Trueness, 3D deviation, time and cost comparisons between milled and 3D-printed resin single crowns. Eur J Prosthodont Restor Dent. 2021;
10. The most common 3D file formats [Internet]. All3DP. 2019 [cited 2021 Oct 5]. Available from: https://all3dp.com/3d-file-format-3d-files-3d-printer-3d-cad-vrml-stl-obj/.
11. Professional 3D printing made accessible | Ultimaker [Internet]. ultimaker.com. [cited 2021 Oct 5]. Available from: https://ultimaker.com/.
12. Netfabb features | Fusion 360 with Netfabb | Autodesk [Internet]. [cited 2021 Oct 5]. Available from: https://www.autodesk.com/products/netfabb/features.
13. PreForm 3D printing software: prepare your models for printing [Internet]. Formlabs. [cited 2021 Oct 5]. Available from: https://formlabs.com/asia/software/.
14. Getting started 3D sprint [Internet]. [cited 2021 Oct 5]. Available from: https://support.3dsystems.com/s/article/3D-Sprint?language=en_US.
15. Timeline of the 3D printing history—ASME [Internet]. [cited 2021 Oct 5]. Available from: https://www.asme.org/topics-resources/content/infographic-the-history-of-3d-printing.
16. History of 3D printing: when was 3D printing invented? [Internet]. All3DP. 2018 [cited 2021 Oct 5]. Available from: https://all3dp.com/2/history-of-3d-printing-when-was-3d-printing-invented/.
17. ISO/ASTM 52900:2015(en), Additive manufacturing—General principles—Terminology [Internet]. [cited 2021 May 2]. Available from: https://www.iso.org/obp/ui/#iso:std:iso-astm:52900:ed-1:v1:en.
18. Directed energy deposition—DED, LENS, EBAM | Make [Internet]. [cited 2021 Oct 5]. Available from: https://make.3dexperience.3ds.com/processes/directed-energy-deposition.
19. Anderson T. Anatomy of a 3D printer: how does a 3D printer work? [Internet]. MatterHackers. [cited 2021 Oct 5]. Available from: https://www.matterhackers.com/articles/anatomy-of-a-3d-printer.
20. Jiang Z, Diggle B, Tan ML, Viktorova J, Bennett CW, Connal LA. Extrusion 3D printing of polymeric materials with advanced properties. Adv Sci. 2020;7(17):2001379.
21. Placone JK, Engler AJ. Recent advances in extrusion-based 3D printing for biomedical applications. Adv Healthc Mater. 2018;7(8):e1701161.
22. Copper 3D | Antibacterial 3D printing—Home [Internet]. Copper 3D | Antibacterial 3D printing. [cited 2021 Oct 5]. Available from: https://copper3d.com/.
23. Antimicrobial materials for 3D printing medical devices [Internet]. 3DHeals. 2020 [cited 2021 Oct 5]. Available from: https://3dheals.com/antimicrobial-materials-for-3d-printing-medical-devices.
24. Gonzalez-Gutierrez J, Cano S, Schuschnigg S, Kukla C, Sapkota J, Holzer C. Additive manufacturing of metallic and ceramic components by the material extrusion of highly-filled polymers: a review and future perspectives. Materials (Basel). 2018;11(5):E840.
25. ExplainingTheFuture.com: 3D printing—Third Edition [Internet]. [cited 2021 May 2]. Available from: https://www.explainingthefuture.com/3dp3e.html.
26. Della Bona A, Cantelli V, Britto VT, Collares KF, Stansbury JW. 3D printing restorative materials using a stereolithographic technique: a systematic review. Dent Mater. 2021;37(2):336–50.
27. Carbon3D introduces CLIP, breakthrough technology for layerless 3D printing [Internet]. Carbon. [cited 2021 Oct 5]. Available from: https://www.carbon3d.com/news/press-releases/carbon3d-introduces-clip-breakthrough-technology-for-layerless-3d-printing/.
28. Kadry H, Wadnap S, Xu C, Ahsan F. Digital light processing (DLP) 3D-printing technology and photoreactive polymers in fabrication of modified-release tablets. Eur J Pharm Sci. 2019;135:60–7.
29. Mayer F, Ryklin D, Wacker I, Curticean R, Čalkovský M, Niemeyer A, et al. 3D two-photon microprinting of nanoporous architectures. Adv Mater. 2020;32(32):e2002044.
30. Correa DS, Tayalia P, Cosendey G, dos Santos DS, Aroca RF, Mazur E, et al. Two-photon polymerization for fabricating structures containing the biopolymer chitosan. J Nanosci Nanotechnol. 2009;9(10):5845–9.
31. Skoog SA, Nguyen AK, Kumar G, Zheng J, Goering PL, Koroleva A, et al. Two-photon polymerization of 3-D zirconium oxide hybrid scaffolds for long-term stem cell growth. Biointerphases. 2014;9(2):029014.
32. Bai Y, Williams CB. The effect of inkjetted nanoparticles on metal part properties in binder jetting additive manufacturing. Nanotechnology. 2018;29(39):395706.
33. Gülcan O, Günaydın K, Tamer A. The state of the art of material jetting-a critical review. Polymers. 2021;13(16):2829.

34. Hong D, Chou D-T, Velikokhatnyi OI, Roy A, Lee B, Swink I, et al. Binder-jetting 3D printing and alloy development of new biodegradable Fe-Mn-Ca/Mg alloys. Acta Biomater. 2016;45:375–86.
35. Meenashisundaram GK, Xu Z, Nai MLS, Lu S, Ten JS, Wei J. Binder jetting additive manufacturing of high porosity 316L stainless steel metal foams. Materials (Basel). 2020;13(17):E3744.
36. Na O, Kim K, Lee H, Lee H. Printability and setting time of CSA cement with Na2SiO3 and gypsum for binder jetting 3D printing. Materials (Basel). 2021;14(11):2811.
37. Păcurar R, Berce P, Nemeş O, Băilă D-I, Stan DS, Oarcea A, et al. Cast iron parts obtained in ceramic molds produced by binder jetting 3D printing-morphological and mechanical characterization. Materials (Basel). 2021;14(16):4502.
38. Goguta L, Lungeanu D, Negru R, Birdeanu M, Jivanescu A, Sinescu C. Selective laser sintering versus selective laser melting and computer aided design–computer aided manufacturing in double crowns retention. J Prosthodont Res. 2021;65(3):371–8.
39. Wang Z, Ummethala R, Singh N, Tang S, Suryanarayana C, Eckert J, et al. Selective laser melting of aluminum and its alloys. Materials (Basel). 2020;13(20):E4564.
40. Bartolomeu F, Costa MM, Alves N, Miranda G, Silva FS. Selective laser melting of Ti6Al4V sub-millimetric cellular structures: prediction of dimensional deviations and mechanical performance. J Mech Behav Biomed Mater. 2021;113:104123.
41. Bulina NV, Baev SG, Makarova SV, Vorobyev AM, Titkov AI, Bessmeltsev VP, et al. Selective laser melting of hydroxyapatite: perspectives for 3D printing of bioresorbable ceramic implants. Materials (Basel). 2021;14(18):5425.
42. Jamshidi P, Aristizabal M, Kong W, Villapun V, Cox SC, Grover LM, et al. Selective laser melting of Ti-6Al-4V: the Impact of post-processing on the tensile, fatigue and biological properties for medical implant applications. Materials (Basel). 2020;13(12):E2813.
43. Ginestra P, Ferraro RM, Zohar-Hauber K, Abeni A, Giliani S, Ceretti E. Selective laser melting and electron beam melting of Ti6Al4V for orthopedic applications: a comparative study on the applied building direction. Materials (Basel). 2020;13(23):E5584.
44. Galati M, Minetola P, Rizza G. Surface roughness characterisation and analysis of the electron beam melting (EBM) process. Materials (Basel). 2019;12(13):E2211.
45. Tamayo JA, Riascos M, Vargas CA, Baena LM. Additive manufacturing of Ti6Al4V alloy via electron beam melting for the development of implants for the biomedical industry. Heliyon. 2021;7(5):e06892.
46. Benedetti M, Torresani E, Leoni M, Fontanari V, Bandini M, Pederzolli C, et al. The effect of post-sintering treatments on the fatigue and biological behavior of Ti-6Al-4V ELI parts made by selective laser melting. J Mech Behav Biomed Mater. 2017;71:295–306.
47. Directed energy deposition—an overview | ScienceDirect Topics [Internet]. [cited 2021 Oct 5]. Available from: https://www.sciencedirect.com/topics/materials-science/directed-energy-deposition.
48. Tao Y, Yin Q, Li P. An additive manufacturing method using large-scale wood inspired by laminated object manufacturing and plywood technology. Polymers. 2020;13(1):E144.
49. Tanabe G, Churei H, Wada T, Takahashi H, Uo M, Ueno T. The influence of temperature on sheet lamination process when fabricating mouthguard on dental thermoforming machine. J Oral Sci. 2020;62(1):23–7.
50. AM 101: Ultrasonic Additive Manufacturing | Additive Manufacturing [Internet]. [cited 2021 Oct 5]. Available from: https://www.additivemanufacturing.media/articles/am-101-ultrasonic-additive-manufacturing.
51. Bournias-Varotsis A, Friel RJ, Harris RA, Engstrøm DS. Ultrasonic Additive Manufacturing as a form-then-bond process for embedding electronic circuitry into a metal matrix. J Manuf Process. 2018;32:664–75.
52. Zeller A-N, Neuhaus M-T, Fresenborg S, Zimmerer RM, Jehn P, Spalthoff S, et al. Accurate and cost-effective mandibular biomodels: a standardized evaluation of 3D-Printing via fused layer deposition modeling on soluble support structures. J Stomatol Oral Maxillofac Surg. 2021;122(4):355–60.
53. Guide to post-processing and finishing SLA 3D prints [Internet]. [cited 2021 Oct 5]. Available from: https://formlabs.com/asia/blog/post-processing-and-finishing-sla-prints/.
54. 3D print post processing—ultimate guide—16 ways [Internet]. [cited 2021 Oct 5]. Available from: https://bigrep.com/post-processing/.
55. Chandki R, Kala M. Natural tooth versus implant: a key to treatment planning. J Oral Implantol. 2012;38(1):95–100.
56. Pjetursson BE, Heimisdottir K. Dental implants—are they better than natural teeth? Eur J Oral Sci. 2018;126(Suppl 1):81–7.
57. Londono J, Tadros M, Salgueiro M, Baker PS. Digital design and 3D printing of an implant-supported prosthetic stent for protecting complete arch soft tissue grafts around dental implants: a dental technique. J Prosthet Dent. 2018;120(6):801–4.
58. Kim T, Lee S, Kim GB, Hong D, Kwon J, Park J-W, et al. Accuracy of a simplified 3D-printed implant surgical guide. J Prosthet Dent. 2020;124(2):195–201.e2.
59. Yeung M, Abdulmajeed A, Carrico CK, Deeb GR, Bencharit S. Accuracy and precision of 3D-printed implant surgical guides with different

implant systems: an in vitro study. J Prosthet Dent. 2020;123(6):821–8.
60. Dong T, Wang X, Xia L, Yuan L, Ye N, Fang B. Accuracy of different tooth surfaces on 3D printed dental models: orthodontic perspective. BMC Oral Health. 2020;20(1):340.
61. Maria R, Tan MY, Wong KM, Lee BCH, Chia VAP, Tan KBC. Accuracy of implant analogs in 3D printed resin models. J Prosthodont. 2021;30(1):57–64.
62. Rungrojwittayakul O, Kan JY, Shiozaki K, Swamidass RS, Goodacre BJ, Goodacre CJ, et al. Accuracy of 3D printed models created by two technologies of printers with different designs of model base. J Prosthodont. 2020;29(2):124–8.
63. Sherman SL, Kadioglu O, Currier GF, Kierl JP, Li J. Accuracy of digital light processing printing of 3-dimensional dental models. Am J Orthod Dentofac Orthop. 2020;157(3):422–8.
64. Chaturvedi S, Alqahtani NM, Addas MK, Alfarsi MA. Marginal and internal fit of provisional crowns fabricated using 3D printing technology. Technol Health Care. 2020;28(6):635–42.
65. Mai H-N, Lee K-B, Lee D-H. Fit of interim crowns fabricated using photopolymer-jetting 3D printing. J Prosthet Dent. 2017;118(2):208–15.
66. Zimmermann M, Ender A, Egli G, Özcan M, Mehl A. Fracture load of CAD/CAM-fabricated and 3D-printed composite crowns as a function of material thickness. Clin Oral Investig. 2019;23(6):2777–84.
67. Methani MM, Revilla-León M, Zandinejad A. The potential of additive manufacturing technologies and their processing parameters for the fabrication of all-ceramic crowns: a review. J Esthet Restor Dent. 2020;32(2):182–92.
68. Matinlinna JP, Choi AH, Tsoi JK-H. Bonding promotion of resin composite to silica-coated zirconia implant surface using a novel silane system. Clin Oral Implants Res. 2013;24(3):290–6.
69. Han A, Tsoi JK-H, Matinlinna JP, Chen Z. Influence of grit-blasting and hydrofluoric acid etching treatment on surface characteristics and biofilm formation on zirconia. Coatings. 2017;7(8):130.
70. Han A, Tsoi JKH, Matinlinna JP, Zhang Y, Chen Z. Effects of different sterilization methods on surface characteristics and biofilm formation on zirconia in vitro. Dent Mater. 2018;34(2):272–81.
71. Dehurtevent M, Robberecht L, Hornez J-C, Thuault A, Deveaux E, Béhin P. Stereolithography: a new method for processing dental ceramics by additive computer-aided manufacturing. Dent Mater. 2017;33(5):477–85.
72. Control of the cross section geometry of extruded dental porcelain slurries for rapid prototyping applications [Internet]. [cited 2021 Oct 5]. Available from: https://repositories.lib.utexas.edu/handle/2152/78543.
73. Tai J, Gan HY, Liang YN, Lok BK.. Control of droplet formation in inkjet printing Using Ohnesorge number category: materials and processes. In: 2008 10th Electronics packaging technology conference. 2008. p. 761–6.
74. Edelmann A, Riedel L, Hellmann R. Realization of a dental framework by 3D printing in material cobalt-chromium with superior precision and fitting accuracy. Materials (Basel). 2020;13(23):E5390.
75. Revilla León M, Klemm IM, García-Arranz J, Özcan M. 3D metal printing—additive manufacturing technologies for frameworks of implant-borne fixed dental prosthesis. Eur J Prosthodont Restor Dent. 2017;25(3):143–7.
76. Presotto AGC, Barão VAR, Bhering CLB, Mesquita MF. Dimensional precision of implant-supported frameworks fabricated by 3D printing. J Prosthet Dent. 2019;122(1):38–45.
77. Thakur J, Parlani S, Shivakumar S, Jajoo K. Accuracy of marginal fit of an implant-supported framework fabricated by 3D printing versus subtractive manufacturing technique: a systematic review and meta-analysis. J Prosthet Dent. 2021;S0022-3913(21):00274–2.
78. Sumida T, Otawa N, Kamata YU, Kamakura S, Mtsushita T, Kitagaki H, et al. Custom-made titanium devices as membranes for bone augmentation in implant treatment: clinical application and the comparison with conventional titanium mesh. J Craniomaxillofac Surg. 2015;43(10):2183–8.
79. Inoue K, Nakajima Y, Omori M, Suwa Y, Kato-Kogoe N, Yamamoto K, et al. Reconstruction of the alveolar bone using bone augmentation with selective laser melting titanium mesh sheet: a report of 2 cases. Implant Dent. 2018;27(5):602–7.
80. Surovas A. A digital workflow for modeling of custom dental implants. 3D Print Med. 2019;5(1):9.
81. Westover B. Three-dimensional custom-root replicate tooth dental implants. Oral Maxillofac Surg Clin N Am. 2019;31(3):489–96.
82. Matinlinna JP, Tsoi JK-H, de Vries J, Busscher HJ. Characterization of novel silane coatings on titanium implant surfaces. Clin Oral Implants Res. 2013;24(6):688–97.
83. Villard N, Seneviratne C, Tsoi JKH, Heinonen M, Matinlinna J. Candida albicans aspects of novel silane system-coated titanium and zirconia implant surfaces. Clin Oral Implants Res. 2015;26(3):332–41.
84. Alcheikh A, Pavon-Djavid G, Helary G, Petite H, Migonney V, Anagnostou F. PolyNaSS grafting on titanium surfaces enhances osteoblast differentiation and inhibits Staphylococcus aureus adhesion. J Mater Sci Mater Med. 2013;24(7):1745–54.
85. Divakar DD, Jastaniyah NT, Altamimi HG, Alnakhli YO, Muzaheed n, Alkheraif AA, et al. Enhanced antimicrobial activity of naturally derived bioactive molecule chitosan conjugated silver nanoparticle against dental implant pathogens. Int J Biol Macromol. 2018;108:790–7.
86. Kalberer N, Mehl A, Schimmel M, Müller F, Srinivasan M. CAD-CAM milled versus rapidly prototyped (3D-printed) complete dentures: an

in vitro evaluation of trueness. J Prosthet Dent. 2019;121(4):637–43.
87. Park C, Kee W, Lim H-P, Park S-W. Combining 3D-printed metal and resin for digitally fabricated dentures: a dental technique. J Prosthet Dent. 2020;123(3):389–92.
88. Yoon S-N, Oh KC, Lee SJ, Han J-S, Yoon H-I. Tissue surface adaptation of CAD-CAM maxillary and mandibular complete denture bases manufactured by digital light processing: a clinical study. J Prosthet Dent. 2020;124(6):682–9.
89. Yang Y, Yang Z, Lin W-S, Chen L, Tan J. Digital duplication and 3D printing for implant overdenture fabrication. J Prosthodont. 2021;30(S2):139–42.
90. Prpić V, Schauperl Z, Ćatić A, Dulčić N, Čimić S. Comparison of mechanical properties of 3D-printed, CAD/CAM, and conventional denture base materials. J Prosthodont. 2020;29(6):524–8.
91. Kumar H, Kim K. Stereolithography 3D bioprinting. Methods Mol Biol Clifton NJ. 2020;2140: 93–108.
92. Nakamura M, Ogura R, Yoshiike N, Teraguchi H. Additive organ manufacturing: challenges to produce organs by biomedical engineering. Organ Biol. 2017;24(2):217–22.
93. Mir TA, Nakamura M. 3D-BioPrinting: towards the era of manufacturing human organs as spare parts for healthcare and medicine. Tissue Eng Part B Rev. 2017;23
94. Mironov V, Prestwich G, Forgacs G. Bioprinting living structures. J Mater Chem. 2007;17
95. Organovo: bioprinting tissue to speed up drug development [Internet]. Technology and Operations Management. [cited 2021 Oct 5]. Available from: https://digital.hbs.edu/platform-rctom/submission/organovo-bioprinting-tissue-to-speed-up-drug-development/.
96. Tong A, Pham QL, Abatemarco P, Mathew A, Gupta D, Iyer S, et al. Review of low-cost 3D bioprinters: state of the market and observed future trends. SLAS Technol Transl Life Sci Innov. 2021;26(4):333–66.
97. Perez-Valle A, Del Amo C, Andia I. Overview of current advances in extrusion bioprinting for skin applications. Int J Mol Sci. 2020;21(18):E6679.
98. O'Connell CD, Konate S, Onofrillo C, Kapsa R, Baker C, Duchi S, et al. Free-form co-axial bioprinting of a gelatin methacryloyl bio-ink by direct in situ photo-crosslinking during extrusion. Bioprinting. 2020;19:e00087.
99. Li L, Tang Q, Wang A, Chen Y. Regrowing a tooth: in vitro and in vivo approaches. Curr Opin Cell Biol. 2019;61:126–31.
100. Capellato P, Camargo SEA, Sachs D. Biological response to nanosurface modification on metallic biomaterials. Curr Osteoporos Rep. 2020;
101. Kuang X, Wu J, Chen K, Zhao Z, Ding Z, Hu F, et al. Grayscale digital light processing 3D printing for highly functionally graded materials. Sci Adv. 2019;5(5):eaav5790.
102. Astaneh SH, Faverani LP, Sukotjo C, Takoudis CG. Atomic layer deposition on dental materials: processing conditions and surface functionalization to improve physical, chemical, and clinical properties - a review. Acta Biomater. 2020;
103. Dutta B, Froes FH. Chapter 3—additive manufacturing technology. In: Dutta B, Froes FH, editors. Additive manufacturing of titanium alloys [Internet]. Butterworth-Heinemann; 2016. [cited 2021 Oct 5]. p. 25–40. Available from: https://www.sciencedirect.com/science/article/pii/B9780128047828000033.
104. Kim J-H, Kim M-Y, Knowles JC, Choi S, Kang H, Park S-H, et al. Mechanophysical and biological properties of a 3D-printed titanium alloy for dental applications. Dent Mater. 2020;36(7):945–58.

GPSR Compliance

The European Union's (EU) General Product Safety Regulation (GPSR) is a set of rules that requires consumer products to be safe and our obligations to ensure this.

If you have any concerns about our products, you can contact us on ProductSafety@springernature.com

In case Publisher is established outside the EU, the EU authorized representative is:

Springer Nature Customer Service Center GmbH
Europaplatz 3
69115 Heidelberg, Germany

Batch number: 10731387

Printed by Printforce, the Netherlands